Management of the Menopause

5th edition

Margaret Rees, John Stevenson, Sally Hope, Serge Rozenberg
and Santiago Palacios

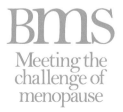

BMS
Meeting the
challenge of
menopause

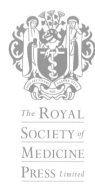

The ROYAL
SOCIETY of
MEDICINE
PRESS Limited

© 2009 Royal Society of Medicine Press Ltd and British Menopause Society Publications Ltd

Published by the Royal Society of Medicine Press Ltd   and   British Menopause Society Publications Ltd
1 Wimpole Street, London W1G 0AE, UK   4-6 Eton Place, Marlow, SL9 2QA, UK
Tel: +44 (0)20 7290 2921   Tel: +44 (0)1628 890199
Fax: +44 (0)20 7290 2929   Fax: +44 (0)1628 474024
Email: publishing@rsm.ac.uk   Email: admin@thebms.org.uk
Website: www.rsmpress.co.uk   Website: www.thebms.org.uk

British Library Cataloguing in Publication Data
A catalogue record for this book is available from the British Library
ISBN 978-1-85315-884-1

Distribution in Europe and Rest of World:
Marston Book Services Ltd
PO Box 269
Abingdon
Oxon OX14 4YN, UK
Tel: +44 (0)1235 465500
Fax: +44 (0)1235 465555
Email: direct.order@marston.co.uk

Distribution in the USA and Canada:
Royal Society of Medicine Press Ltd
c/o BookMasters, Inc.
30 Amberwood Parkway
Ashland, Ohio 44805, USA
Tel: +1- 00 247 6553 / +1 800 266 5564
Email: order@bookmasters.com

Distribution in Australia and New Zealand:
Elsevier Australia
30–52 Smidmore Street
Marrickville NSW 2204, Australia
Tel: +61 2 9349 5811
Fax: +61 2 9349 5911
Email: service@elsevier.com.au

Designed and typeset by Saxon Graphics Ltd, Derby
Printed and bound by Bell & Bain Ltd, Glasgow

Contents

About the authors

Margaret Rees MA DPhil FRCOG is a Reader in Reproductive Medicine at the Nuffield Department of Obstetrics and Gynaecology, University of Oxford, and a Visiting Professor at the University of Glasgow and the Karolinska Institute. Her areas of interest are menopause and menstrual disorders and she has contributed towards over 300 publications. In both areas she has undertaken both laboratory and clinical research. She has authored and edited 20 books, two of which were highly commended in BMA Book Awards. She is the Editor-in-Chief of *Maturitas* and former Editor-in-Chief of *Menopause International*. She is also a Council member of the Committee of Publication Ethics (COPE). In 2006 she was awarded the Egon Diczfalusy Medal by the Karolinska Institute in recognition of her international profile in reproductive medicine.

John Stevenson FRCP FESC MFSEM is a Reader in Metabolic Medicine at the National Heart and Lung Institute, Imperial College London, and Consultant Physician at the Royal Brompton Hospital, London, where he jointly runs the UK's first Female Heart Disease Clinic. He has contributed towards over 370 journal articles and book publications, including 10 textbooks. He is Chairman of the charity Women's Health Concern, Executive Committee Member of the British Menopause Society, Fellow of the European Society of Cardiology, Foundation Member of the Faculty of Sports and Exercise Medicine (UK), and is one of the editors of *Maturitas*.

Sally Hope FRCGP DRCOG is a General Practitioner in Woodstock, Oxfordshire and an Honorary Research Fellow in Women's Health at the University of Oxford. She is a founding member of the Primary Care Group in Gynaecology and is the Royal College of General Practitioners' representative for the National Institute for Health and Clinical Excellence guideline group on osteoporosis. She has authored and contributed to major textbooks on women's health and was formerly Deputy Editor of *Menopause International*.

Serge Rozenberg MD PhD is a Clinical Professor of Obstetrics and Gynaecology at the Université Libre de Bruxelles, Belgium. He is in charge of the menopause and osteoporosis unit at the CHU St Pierre, and is a recognized authority in women's health. He has published more than 100 articles in international peer-reviewed journals on topics such as women's health, menopause, osteoporosis and reproductive endocrinology. He is on the editorial board of several international journals and has received several awards and grants for his research. He is also currently the secretary of EMAS and one of the editors of *Maturitas*.

Santiago Palacios is Director of the Instituto Palacios de Salud y Medicina de la Mujer (Palacios Institute of Woman's Health), in Madrid, Spain. He is President of the European Foundation for Womean and Health, and Chairman of the Council of Affiliated Menopause Societies (CAMS). In 1989, Dr Palacios founded the first Spanish Unit devoted to the advancement of information on menopause at the Foundation Jimenez Diaz. His most important research areas are menopause, osteoporosis and female sexual dysfunction. He has contributed towards more than 300 publications in books and journal articles on women's health. He is a member of several Menopause Societies in Europe and Latin America, and has received many awards in recognition of his international profile.

Foreword

The fifth edition of *Management of the Menopause* is truly international, and hence the two authors of the Foreword, Louis Keith and Michael Cust, provide a US and a UK view respectively.

Louis Keith

When Margaret Rees sent me the contents of this book with the idea of my writing a Foreword to it, I experienced a double-sided sense of *déjà vu*. On the one hand, my mind raced back to my days as an intern at the Cook County Hospital in Chicago, when, in 1960, Professor M Edward Davis of the University of Chicago was expounding loudly to all who would listen regarding the treatment of the menopause. It was a short and simple message – two words in fact, 'estrogens forever'. On the other hand, I rushed to peruse the table of contents of *Management of the Menopause* and found far more than two words – to be exact, 14 chapters.

What does this expansion tell us? Simplistically, it details the expansion of the knowledge base about an important phase of women's lives and the growing numbers of women who will live 30–40 years or more beyond it. This is something that was not a major consideration for the medical profession and governmental agencies when Professor Davis was making light of it. More realistically, however, this book details how the profession has come to regard what was a rather old-fashioned way of looking at a specific point in women's lives; that is, their 'change in life'.

In truth, *Management of the Menopause* could have droned on for 1000 or more pages, but the authors knew that this is not what busy healthcare professionals want or are looking for. Such books abound, but they do not fit in one's coat pocket; this one does and that is its appeal. Is there more to say than that which is contained in the chapters? Of course there is, and every chapter is supplemented with a long, up-to-date list of additional resources that take the place of traditional references at the end of each sentence. That having been said, what is there for every reader is a great start, and certainly enough to go to the consulting rooms or clinics, answer questions, and prescribe therapies that are useful to the patient. Such therapies, advice and suggestions will be of great use to all who take care of menopausal patients and are not restricted to gynaecologists. Thus, it is essential reading for hospital or primary-care physicians, nurses or allied health professionals. The book's great value is that it is not intimidating to anyone at any level of training and that it has been extensively revised since the previous edition in 2006. This edition has all the hallmarks of success that graced its predecessors.

For any busy clinician, a textbook should fulfil certain criteria. It needs to be interesting, relevant, readable and current, and to provide information that is easy to find. This fifth edition of *Management of the Menopause* does all of these in a format and style that invite the reader to learn more.

Louis Keith MD PhD ScD (Hon)
Emeritus Professor of Obstetrics and Gynecology
Northwestern University, Chicago, USA

Michael Cust

This was a formidable undertaking, to build on the previous editions and include all of the rapid advances in our knowledge of the menopause and its treatment. This latest edition has expanded from 12 chapters in 2006 to 14, such is the breadth of our knowledge now.

Within these chapters, all aspects of the menopause are covered. Starting with the physiology, symptoms and assessment of the woman, it continues with detailed sections on hormonal and non-hormonal treatments. There are chapters with advice about how the menopause and hormones affect benign and malignant diseases. One chapter is devoted to women with premature ovarian failure, a group who were particularly hard-hit by some of the misinformation about hormone therapy since the Women's Health Initiative study of 2002.

Although written under the auspices of the British Menopause Society, the content of the book is universal, and the authors are international. Clinicians from all over the world will find the advice relevant to their patients. It will suit all grades of reader, from the early trainee to the experienced specialist. For anyone involved in looking after women around the time of the menopause, it will no doubt prove to be an invaluable guide, to be kept close at hand in the consulting room.

Mike Cust MB BS FRCOG
Consultant Obstetrician and Gynaecologist
Derby City General Hospital, UK

Preface

Women's health is increasingly recognized as a global health priority. With the expanding elderly female population, the long-term complications of ageing and oestrogen deficiency present an enormous problem in terms of morbidity, mortality and economic burden. Thus, managing postreproductive health is becoming a key issue for all health professionals, not just gynaecologists. Publication of large, randomized trials and observational studies in specific populations, and the reactions to these by the media have generated confusion in both lay and professional circles about the best course to take.

The aim of the book is to provide a practical, unbiased and non-promotional international guide for all health professionals dealing with menopausal and postmenopausal women. The authors are international, being based in the UK, Belgium and Spain. Advice has also been sought from Karin Schenck-Gustafsson at the Karolinska Institute in Sweden, Martin Oehler at the University of Adelaide in Australia, and Victor Henderson at Stanford University in the USA, as well as members of the British Menopause Society Council. The evidence base, where available, is presented. This fifth edition has been substantially revised and updated from the fourth, published in 2006. Previous editions have been cited by other organizations such as the Council of Affiliated Menopause Societies, and they form the template for menopause training modules for health professionals.

The book is in four sections: the menopause and postmenopausal health; assessment and investigations; management strategies and women with special needs – such as those with a premature menopause. With regard to management strategies, both oestrogen and non-oestrogen-based treatments and their relative merits are discussed. Evidence regarding alternative and complementary therapies, as well as diet and lifestyle issues, is also presented. The book therefore provides an integrated approach to postreproductive health.

Margaret Rees
John Stevenson
Sally Hope
Serge Rozenberg
Santiago Palacios

THE MENOPAUSE AND POSTMENOPAUSAL HEALTH

1 The menopause: physiology and definitions

Introduction

The menopause is defined as the cessation of the menstrual cycle and is caused by ovarian failure. The term is derived from the Greek *menos*, meaning month, and *pausos*, meaning an ending. The median age at which the menopause occurs is 52 years.

Worldwide, increasing life expectancy and decreasing fertility rates mean that the number of older people is projected to grow considerably in absolute and relative terms. Between 1950 and 2007, the percentage of people aged 65 and older increased from 5% to 7% worldwide. Europe and Japan have led the way with 15% or more aged 65 or over, followed by North America, Australia and New Zealand (10–14%). However, older people are no more than 5% of the inhabitants of many developing countries and by 2050 are expected to be 19% of Latin America's population and 18% of Asia's.

Furthermore, the United Nations Population Division world population projections to 2300 estimate that, between 2100 and 2300, the proportion of world population 65 years and older will increase by one-third (from 24% to 32%); the proportion 80 years and older will double (from 8.5% to 17%); and the proportion 100 years and older will increase by nine times (from 0.2% to 1.8%).

Thus, the menopause can now be considered to be a midlife event.

Definitions

Various definitions are in use and are detailed below.

- **Menopause** is the permanent cessation of menstruation that results from loss of ovarian follicular activity. Natural menopause is recognized to have occurred after 12 consecutive months of amenorrhoea for which no other obvious pathological or physiological cause is present. Menopause occurs with the final menstrual period and thus is known with certainty only in retrospect one year after the event. No adequate biological marker exists.

- **Perimenopause** includes the period beginning with the first clinical, biological and endocrinological features of the approaching menopause, such as vasomotor symptoms and menstrual irregularity, and ends 12 months after the last menstrual period.

- **Premenopause** is a term often used ambiguously to refer to the 1–2 years immediately before the menopause or to the whole of the reproductive period before the menopause. Currently, this term is recommended to be used in the latter sense, encompassing the entire reproductive period from menarche to the final menstrual period.

- **Postmenopause** should be defined from the final menstrual period regardless of whether the menopause was induced or spontaneous. Surgical menopause is timed precisely, but, as noted above, the time of natural menopause can only be determined retrospectively after a period of 12 months of spontaneous amenorrhoea.

- **Menopausal transition** is the period of time before the final menstrual period, when variability in the menstrual cycle usually is increased.

- **Climacteric** is the phase encompassing the transition from the reproductive state to the non-reproductive state. The menopause itself thus is a specific event that occurs during the climacteric – just as the menarche is a specific event that occurs during puberty.

- **Climacteric syndrome** – the climacteric is sometimes but not always associated with symptoms. When this occurs, the term 'climacteric syndrome' may be used.

- **Induced menopause** is the cessation of menstruation that follows surgical removal of both ovaries or iatrogenic ablation of ovarian function by chemotherapy, radiotherapy or treatment with gonadotrophin-releasing hormone analogues. In the absence of surgery, induced menopause may be permanent or temporary.

Determinants of the age of menopause

The age at menopause may be determined by genetic and environmental factors. Growth restriction in late gestation, low weight gain in infancy and starvation in early childhood may be associated with an earlier menopause. It also occurs earlier in women with Down's syndrome and in smokers. However, being breastfed, higher childhood cognitive ability, and increasing parity delay the age of menopause. Japanese race and ethnicity may be associated with later age of natural menopause.

Ovarian function

The main steroid hormones produced by the ovary are oestradiol, progesterone and testosterone. In premenopausal women, ovarian function is controlled by the two pituitary gonadotrophins: follicle-stimulating hormone (FSH) and luteinizing hormone (LH). Follicle-stimulating hormone itself is controlled primarily by the pulsatile secretion of hypothalamic gonadotrophin-releasing hormone (GnRH) and is modulated by the negative feedback of oestradiol and progesterone and the ovarian peptide

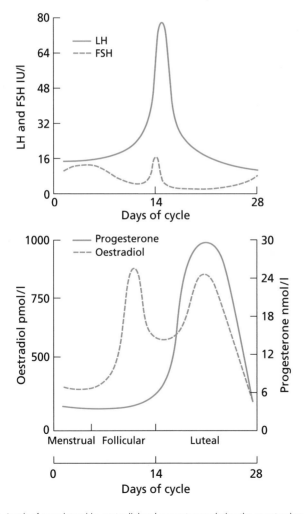

Figure 1.1 Levels of gonadatrophin, oestradiol and progesterone during the menstural cycle

inhibin B. Luteinizing hormone is under the principal control of GnRH, with negative feedback control from oestradiol and progesterone for most of the cycle; positive oestradiol feedback generates the mid-cycle surge in levels of LH that triggers ovulation (Figure 1.1).

Each ovary receives a finite endowment of oocytes, the numbers of which are maximal at 20–28 weeks of intrauterine life. From mid-gestation onwards, a logarithmic reduction in these germ cells occurs until, about 50 years later, the stock of oocytes is depleted. The ovary gradually becomes less responsive to gonadotrophins several years before menstruation stops. This results in a reduction in production of oestrogen and an increase in levels of gonadotrophins. There is thus a gradual increase in circulating levels of FSH and later of LH, and a decrease in levels of oestradiol and inhibin B. Levels of FSH fluctuate markedly from premenopausal to postmenopausal values on virtually a daily basis during the menopausal transition (Figure 1.2). Their diagnostic use thus is severely limited (see Chapter 5). These changes in circulating levels of hormones frequently occur with ovulatory cycles. As ovarian unresponsiveness becomes more marked, cycles tend to become anovulatory, and complete failure of follicular development eventually occurs. Production of oestradiol is no longer sufficient to stimulate the endometrium, leading to amenorrhoea, with levels of FSH and LH now persistently elevated. Levels of FSH of >30 IU/l are generally considered to be in the postmenopausal range.

The ovaries are an important source of testosterone, which is hydroxylated to dihydrotestosterone. Testosterone also can be aromatized to oestradiol. Precursor hormones, such as androstenedione and dehydroepiandrosterone (DHEA), are produced in the ovaries and the adrenals, and both possess a less potent androgenic effect than testosterone. By the time women reach their mid-40s, mean circulating levels of testosterone, androstenedione,

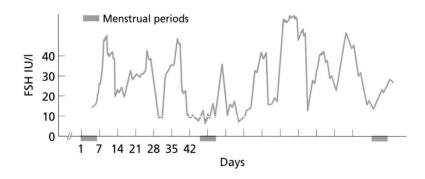

Figure 1.2 Levels of follicle-stimulating hormone during the menopause

Final menstrual period (FMP)

Stages:	−5	−4	−3	−2	−1	0	+1	+2
Terminology:	Reproductive			Menopausal transition			Postmenopause	
	Early	Peak	Late	Early	Late*		Early*	Late
				Perimenopause				
Duration of stages:	Variable			Variable		a) 1 year / b) 4 yrs		Until demise
Menstrual cycles:	Variable to regular	Regular		Variable cycle length (>7 days different from normal)	≥2 skipped cycles and an interval of amenorrhoea (≥60 days)	Amen = 12 mos	None	
Endocrine:	normal FSH		↑FSH	↑FSH	↑FSH		↑FSH	↑FSH

*Stages most likely to be characterized by vasomotor symptoms   ↑ = elevated

Figure 1.3 STRAW staging system for reproductive ageing. Reprinted from Soules MR et al (2001), with permission from American Society for Reproductive Medicine

DHEA and the sulphate product (DHEA-S) are approximately half those of women in their 20s. Menopausal status does not affect levels of androgens in women aged 45–54 years, however, and the postmenopausal ovary seems to be an ongoing site of testosterone production. Low circulating levels of androgens have been proposed to be associated with low sexual desire; however, no level of a single androgen is predictive of low sexual function in women.

Stages of reproductive ageing

A staging system that uses the final or last menstrual period (FMP) as the anchor to describe reproductive ageing was proposed by the Stages of Reproductive Aging Workshop (STRAW). In this system, five stages precede and two stages follow the FMP. Stages –5 to –3 encompass the reproductive interval, stages –2 and –1 are the menopausal transition and stages 1 and 2 are the postmenopause (Figure 1.3). After menarche (stage –5), it usually takes several years for regular menstrual cycles to become established. Menstrual periods should then occur every 21–35 days for a number of years (stages –4 and –3). A woman's menstrual cycles remain regular in stage –2 (early menopausal transition), but the duration changes by 7 days or more (cycles are now every 24 days instead of every 31 days). Stage –1 (late menopausal transition) is characterized by two or more missed periods and at least one intermenstrual interval of 60 days or more. Stages +1 (early) and +2 (late) encompass the postmenopause. The early postmenopause is defined as 5 years since the FMP and the late postmenopause thereafter until death. Progression through the STRAW stages is associated with elevations in serum FSH, LH, and oestradiol and decreases in luteal phase progesterone.

Further reading

Demography

Cassou B, Mandereau L, Aegerter P, Touranchet A, Derriennic F. Work-related factors associated with age at natural menopause in a generation of French gainfully employed women. *Am J Epidemiol* 2007;**166**:429–38.

Elias SG, van Noord PA, Peeters PH, *et al.* Caloric restriction reduces age at menopause: the effect of the 1944–1945 Dutch famine. *Menopause* 2003;**10**: 399–405.

Gold EB, Bromberger J, Crawford S, *et al.* Factors associated with age at natural menopause in a multiethnic sample of midlife women. *Am J Epidemiol* 2001;**153**: 865–74.

Gosden RG, Treloar SA, Martin NG, *et al.* Prevalence of premature ovarian failure in monozygotic and dizygotic twins. *Hum Reprod* 2007;**22**:610–15.

Kinsella KG. Future longevity-demographic concerns and consequences. *J Am Geriatr Soc* 2005;**53**(9 Suppl):S299–303.

Michel JP, Newton JL, Kirkwood TB. Medical challenges of improving the quality of a longer life. *JAMA* 2008;**299**:688–90.

Mishra G, Hardy R, Kuh D. Are the effects of risk factors for timing of menopause modified by age? Results from a British birth cohort study. *Menopause* 2007;**14**: 717–24.

Nichols HB, Trentham-Dietz A, Hampton JM, *et al.* From menarche to menopause: trends among US women born from 1912 to 1969. *Am J Epidemiol* 2006;**164**: 1003–11.

Population reference bureau. 2007 World Population Data Sheet. www.prb.org/pdf07/07WPDS_Eng.pdf.

Reynolds RF, Obermeyer CM. Age at natural menopause in Spain and the United States: results from the DAMES project. *Am J Hum Biol* 2005;**17**:331–40.

Seltzer GB, Schupf N, Wu HS. A prospective study of menopause in women with Down's syndrome. *J Intellect Disabil Res* 2001;**45**:1–7.

United Nations Department of Economic and Social Affairs. World Population to 2300. www.un.org/esa/population/publications/longrange2/WorldPop2300final.pdf.

Endocrinology/ovarian function

Bachmann G, Bancroft J, Braunstein G, *et al.* Female androgen insufficiency: the Princeton consensus statement on definition, classification, and assessment. *Fertil Steril* 2002;**77**:660–5.

Burger HG, Hale GE, Dennerstein L, Robertson DM. Cycle and hormone changes during perimenopause: the key role of ovarian function. *Menopause* 2008;**15**: 603–12.

Davis SR, Davison SK, Donath S, *et al.* Circulating androgen levels and self-reported sexual function in women. *JAMA* 2005;**294**:91–6.

Davison S, Bell R, Donath S, *et al.* Androgen levels in adult females: changes with age, menopause and oophorectomy. *J Clin Endocrinol Metab* 2005;**90**:3847–53.

Guay A, Munarriz R, Jacobson J, *et al.* Serum androgen levels in healthy premenopausal women with and without sexual dysfunction: part A. Serum androgen levels in women aged 20–49 years with no complaints of sexual dysfunction. *Int J Impot Res* 2004;**16**:112–20.

Hale GE, Zhao X, Hughes CL, *et al.* Endocrine features of menstrual cycles in middle and late reproductive age and the menopausal transition classified according to the Staging of Reproductive Aging Workshop (STRAW) staging system. *J Clin Endocrinol Metab* 2007;**92**:3060–7.

International Menopause Society. Menopause Terminology. www.imsociety.org/menopause_terminology.html.

Landgren BM, Collins A, Csemiczky G, *et al.* Menopause transition: annual changes in serum hormonal patterns over the menstrual cycle in women during a nine-year period prior to menopause. *J Clin Endocrinol Metab* 2004;**89**:2763–9.

Santoro N, Crawford SL, Lasley WL, *et al*. Factors related to declining luteal function in women during the menopausal transition. *J Clin Endocrinol Metab* 2008;**93**: 1711–21.

Soules MR, Sherman S, Parrott E, *et al*. Executive summary: Stages of Reproductive Aging Workshop (STRAW). *Fertil Steril* 2001;**76**:874–8.

Sowers MR, Eyvazzadeh AD, McConnell D, *et al*. Anti-Müllerian hormone and inhibin B in the definition of ovarian aging and the menopause transition. *J Clin Endocrinol Metab* 2008;**93**:3478–83.

Spencer JB, Klein M, Kumar A, Azziz R. The age-associated decline of androgens in reproductive age and menopausal black and white women. *J Clin Endocrinol Metab* 2007;**92**:4730–3.

2 Menopausal symptoms

Vasomotor symptoms
Sexual dysfunction
Psychological symptoms
Further reading

The change in hormone levels that occurs during the climacteric, particularly the decline in levels of oestrogen, can cause acute menopausal symptoms. About 70% of women in Western cultures experience vasomotor symptoms, such as hot flushes and night sweats. Some women also report psychological symptoms, which can be related to their experience of vasomotor symptoms or menstrual changes or to concurrent life events. These include tiredness, depressed mood, loss of libido, lethargy and arthralgia. Symptom reporting varies between cultures: for example, Japanese women have fewer menopausal complaints than their North American counterparts. Furthermore rural Mayan women living in the Yucatán, Mexico, do not report either hot flushes or night sweats. Symptoms that are most bothersome and troublesome to women during the menopausal transition also vary between cultures. In Japan, the symptom reported more than any other during the perimenopause is shoulder stiffness.

Vasomotor symptoms

Hot flushes and night sweats are the most common symptoms of the menopause, and, although they may begin before periods stop, the prevalence of flushes is highest in the first year after the final menstrual period. Although they are usually present for less than 5 years, some women will continue to flush beyond the age of 60 years. Flushes are episodes of inappropriate heat loss mediated by cutaneous vasodilation over the upper trunk. Sympathetic nervous control of blood flow in the skin is impaired in women with menopausal flushes, in whom reflex constriction to an ice stimulus cannot be elicited. More recently, serotonin and its receptors in the central nervous system have been implicated.

Hot flushes are unpredictable and can occur at any time of the day or night, disturbing normal sleep patterns. Chronically disturbed sleep, in turn, can lead to insomnia, irritability and difficulties with short-term memory and concentration.

Although women with a higher level of education seem to have fewer symptoms, evidence about the effect of exercise is conflicting. Current smoking and high body mass index (BMI) may also predispose a woman to more severe or frequent hot flushes.

Sexual dysfunction

Women increasingly are staying sexually active into their 70s and beyond. Thus, their sexual problems need to be addressed. The term 'female sexual dysfunction' (FSD) is now used. An international classification system was elaborated by the International Consensus Development Conference on Female Sexual Dysfunction (Table 2.1). The categories are not exclusive and can overlap, and one may cause the other. For example, dyspareunia is likely to lead to avoidance of sexual activity, and anticipation of pain leads to lack of arousal, loss of orgasm and increased chance of pain recurring.

Sexual problems in women are common. It has been estimated that they affect about one in two women. Interest in sex declines in both sexes with increasing age, and this change is more pronounced in women. The US National Health and Social Life survey, which was undertaken in people aged 18–59 years, reported that sexual dysfunction is more prevalent in women (43%) than men (31%). Another US study of 1550 women and 1455 men aged 57–85 years found that the prevalence of sexual activity declined with age (73% among respondents who were 57–64 years of age, 53% among respondents who were 65–74 years of age, and 26% among respondents who were 75–85 years of age); women were significantly less likely than men at all ages to report sexual activity. The most prevalent sexual problems among women were low desire (43%), difficulty with vaginal lubrication (39%), and inability to climax (34%).

The underlying reasons for FSD can be divided into hormonal and non-hormonal. Postmenopausal oestrogen deficiency causes atrophic changes. The vaginal mucosa becomes thinner and dry and the vulva and the vaginal walls also become pale and thin and lose their elasticity. Vaginal secretions also decrease, leading to reduced lubrication. Reduced levels of oestrogen can also impair peripheral sensory perception, and women may experience discomfort after contact with the skin by clothes or their partner.

Non-hormonal factors, such as conflict between partners, insomnia, inadequate stimulation, life stress or depression, however, are important contributors to a woman's level of interest in sexual activity. In addition, male sexual problems – for example, loss of libido and erectile difficulties – should not be overlooked.

There has been debate in the literature on the effect of hysterectomy and oophorectomy on sexual function. The effect depends on several factors such as age, preoperative mental health and sexual function, the indications for surgery, the specific procedure being performed, and whether or not oestrogen is used postoperatively. The majority of research on the effects of surgical menopause shows improved psychological wellbeing and sexual function

Table 2.1

Consensus classification system. Adapted from Basson (2000)

Classification	Definition
I **Sexual desire disorders**	
(A) Hypoactive sexual desire disorder (HSDD)	The persistent or recurrent deficiency (or absence) of sexual fantasies/thoughts and/or desire for or receptivity to sexual activity, which causes personal distress
(B) Sexual aversion disorder (SAD)	The persistent or recurrent phobic aversion and avoidance of sexual contact with a sexual partner, which causes personal distress
II **Sexual arousal disorders**	The persistent or recurrent inability to attain or maintain sufficient sexual excitement, causing personal distress, which may be expressed as a lack of subjective excitement, or genital (lubrication/swelling) or other somatic responses
III **Orgasmic disorder**	The persistent or recurrent difficulty, delay in or absence of attaining orgasm after sufficient sexual stimulation and arousal, which causes personal distress
IV **Sexual pain disorders**	
(A) Dyspareunia	The recurrent or persistent genital pain associated with sexual intercourse
(B) Vaginismus	The recurrent or persistent involuntary spasm of the musculature of the outer third of the vagina, which interferes with vaginal penetration and causes personal distress
(C) Non-coital sexual pain disorders	Recurrent or persistent genital pain induced by non-coital sexual stimulation

Each of the categories above is subtyped on the basis of the medical history, physical examination and laboratory tests as: (A) lifelong versus acquired; (B) generalized versus situational or (C) aetiology (organic, psychogenic, mixed or unknown)

after hysterectomy for benign disease. However, women with depression or sexual problems preoperatively are at increased risk of experiencing a worsening of mood and libido postoperatively.

Psychological symptoms

Psychological symptoms, including depressed mood, anxiety, irritability, mood swings, lethargy and lack of energy, have been associated with the menopause. While transition to menopause confers a higher risk of development of depression, most women do not experience major changes in mood during this time.

Prospective epidemiological studies suggest that psychological problems reported during the menopause are likely to be associated with past problems and current life stresses. It is important, therefore, to take account of other factors, such as prior negative mood, history of premenstrual complaints, negative attitudes to ageing or the menopause, and poor health. In the past, the emphasis was on a woman's change of role – for example, the result of an 'empty nest'. In contrast, a wide range of other issues are relevant to women today (Box 2.1).

These physical and life changes can combine to make a woman feel that she is unable to cope. It is essential that these feelings are recognized and that the woman is offered the opportunity to discuss and clarify their possible causes in her particular case. Treatment, if requested, should be targeted to the individual needs of the woman.

Box 2.1

Factors associated with menopausal psychological symptoms

- Ageing parents and their possible increasing dependency
- Death of a parent, relative or friend
- Loss of partner through death, separation or divorce
- Lack of social support
- Educational or marital difficulties of young adult offspring
- Ill health
- Demanding workload or threat of redundancy
- Economic problems
- Coming to terms with ageing in a culture that values youth and fertility
- Vasomotor instability leading to sleep problems and tiredness

Further reading

General symptoms

Alexander JL, Dennerstein L, Woods NF, *et al.* Arthralgias, bodily aches and pains and somatic complaints in midlife women: aetiology, pathophysiology and differential diagnosis. *Expert Rev Neurother* 2007;7(Suppl):S15–26.

Crawford SL. The roles of biologic and nonbiologic factors in cultural differences in vasomotor symptoms measured by surveys. *Menopause* 2007;**14**:725–33.

Melby MK, Lock M, Kaufert P. Culture and symptom reporting at menopause. *Hum Reprod Update* 2005;**11**:495–512.

Vasomotor symptoms

Daley A, MacArthur C, Mutrie N, Stokes-Lampard H. Exercise for vasomotor menopausal symptoms. *Cochrane Database Syst Rev* 2007;**4**:CD006108.

Politi MC, Schleinitz MD, Col NF. Revisiting the duration of vasomotor symptoms of menopause: a meta-analysis. *J Gen Intern Med* 2008;**23**:1507–13.

Smith-DiJulio K, Percival DB, Woods NF, *et al.* Hot flash severity in hormone therapy users/nonusers across the menopausal transition. *Maturitas* 2007;**58**:191–200.

Sievert LL, Obermeyer CM, Price K. Determinants of hot flashes and night sweats. *Ann Hum Biol* 2006;**33**:4–16.

Sturdee DW. The menopausal hot flush – anything new? *Maturitas* 2008;**60**:42–9.

Thurston RC, Sowers MR, Sutton-Tyrrell K, *et al.* Abdominal adiposity and hot flashes among midlife women. *Menopause* 2008;**15**:429–34.

Whiteman MK, Staropoli CA, Langenberg PW, *et al.* Smoking, body mass, and hot flashes in midlife women. *Obstet Gynecol* 2003;**101**:264–72.

Sexual dysfunction

Basson R, Berman J, Burnett A, *et al.* Report of the international consensus development conference on female sexual dysfunction: definitions and classifications. *J Urol* 2000;**163**:888–93.

Beckman N, Waern M, Gustafson D, Skoog I. Secular trends in self reported sexual activity and satisfaction in Swedish 70 year olds: cross sectional survey of four populations, 1971–2001. *BMJ* 2008;**337**:151–4.

Laumann EO, Paik A, Rosen RC. Sexual dysfunction in the United States: prevalence and predictors. *JAMA* 1998;**281**:537–44.

Lindau ST, Schumm LP, Laumann EO, *et al.* A study of sexuality and health among older adults in the United States. *N Engl J Med* 2007;**357**:762–74.

Moreira ED, Glasser DB, Nicolosi A, *et al.*; GSSAB Investigators' Group. Sexual problems and help-seeking behaviour in adults in the United Kingdom and continental Europe. *BJU Int* 2008;**101**:1005–11.

Shifren JL, Avis NE. Surgical menopause: effects on psychological well-being and sexuality. *Menopause* 2007;**14**:586–91.

Smith LJ, Mulhall JP, Deveci S, *et al*. Sex after seventy: a pilot study of sexual function in older persons. *J Sex Med* 2007;4:1247–53.

Wylie KR. Sexuality and the menopause. *J Br Menopause Soc* 2006;12:149–52.

Psychological symptoms

Freeman EW, Sammel MD, Lin H, *et al*. Symptoms in the menopausal transition: hormone and behavioral correlates. *Obstet Gynecol* 2008;111:127–36.

Frey BN, Lord C, Soares CN. Depression during menopausal transition: a review of treatment strategies and pathophysiological correlates. *Menopause Int* 2008;14: 123–8.

Parry BL. Perimenopausal depression. *Am J Psychiatry* 2008;165:23–7.

Vesco KK, Haney EM, Humphrey L, *et al*. Influence of menopause on mood: a systematic review of cohort studies. *Climacteric* 2007;10:448–65.

3 Chronic conditions affecting postmenopausal health

Cardiovascular disease
Obesity
Metabolic syndrome
Osteoporosis
Dementia and cognitive decline
Respiratory problems: chronic obstructive pulmonary disease and
    asthma
Urogenital atrophy and urinary incontinence
Further reading

Women's health is increasingly recognized as a global health priority. With the expanding elderly female population, the long-term complications of ageing and oestrogen deficiency present an enormous problem in terms of morbidity, mortality and economic burden. According to the World Health Organization (WHO), the leading causes of death in women aged over 45 years are cardiovascular disease (CVD) followed by respiratory disease, diabetes and cancer (breast, lung and stomach).

Cardiovascular disease

Coronary heart disease (CHD) and stroke are the primary clinical endpoints of CVD. Cardiovascular disease is the leading cause of death and disability in both sexes in the developed and developing world. Worldwide, CVD is the major cause of death in women, accounting for one-third of all deaths. As CVD increases in prevalence with age, and as women live longer than men, in many countries more women than men die from CVD each year. In the USA, 38.2 million women (34%) are living with CVD. In Europe, CVD is the cause of death in 43% of men and 54% of women. CVD causes more death than all cancers added together (Table 3.1). Stroke is more commonly fatal in women than men (18% vs 11% respectively) whereas deaths from CHD are similar (23% vs 21% respectively). In the UK in 2006, CHD and stroke were responsible for 42,000 (14%) and 34,000 (11%) deaths in women, respectively, out of a total of 297,500. In the USA, CHD causes 27% and stroke 8% of deaths in women.

Table 3.1

Causes of death in men and women

Disease	Men (%)	Women (%)
CAD	21	22
Stroke	11	17
Other CVD	11	15
Cancer	21	17 (breast 3)
Respiratory	7	6
Injuries/poisoning	12	5
Other	17	18

European cardiovascular disease statistics 2008 (latest available year 2005)
CAD, coronary artery disease; CVD, cardiovascular disease

Risk factors

There are various classifications of risk factors for CVD (American Heart Association, SCORE, European Society of Cardiology). The American Heart Association classification for women is shown in Table 3.2.

Non-modifiable risk factors are age, family history and ethnicity. For example, in the USA, mortality from CVD is higher in black than white Americans. Modifiable risk factors are smoking, blood pressure, hyperlipidaemia, diabetes, body weight and abdominal adiposity, and lifestyle factors such as reduced fruit and vegetable intake, alcohol excess, lack of exercise, psychosocial stress.

Smoking

Smoking is one of the principal risk factors for CHD in women. Women under 55 years have a sevenfold increase in relative risk attributable to smoking, and the increase in risk is dose dependent. In addition, smoking multiplies deleteriously with other risk factors.

Blood pressure

Hypertension significantly increases the risk of CHD and stroke. The increase in relative risk is approximately doubled for combined systolic and diastolic hypertension. Isolated systolic hypertension, which is more common in the elderly, is also associated with similar increased risk. The evidence of benefit from treating hypertension is well established.

Target blood pressures are 140/90 mmHg or less in general and 130/80 mmHg or less in those at high risk (diabetes, chronic renal disease) or with established CHD. The benefit curve extends down to 115/75 mmHg, and there is evidence that a more aggressive strategy confers increasing risk reduction.

Table 3.2

Classification of CVD risk in women

Risk status	Criteria
High risk	Established coronary heart disease
	Cerebrovascular disease
	Peripheral artery disease
	Abdominal aortic aneurysm
	End-stage or chronic renal disease
	Diabetes mellitus
	10-year Framingham global risk of >20%*
At risk	≥1 major risk factors for CVD including:
	Cigarette smoking
	Poor diet
	Physical inactivity
	Obesity, especially central adiposity
	Family history of premature CVD (CVD at <55 years of age in male relative and <65 years of age in female relative)
	Hypertension
	Dyslipidaemia
	Evidence of subclinical vascular disease (e.g. coronary calcification)
	Metabolic syndrome
	Poor exercise capacity on treadmill test and/or abnormal heart rate recovery after stopping exercise
Optimal risk	Framingham global risk of <10% and a healthy lifestyle, with no risk factors

CVD, cardiovascular disease
*Or at high risk on the basis of another population-adapted tool used to access global risk. Adapted from Mosca *et al* 2007

Hyperlipidaemia

Elevated cholesterol is associated with an increased risk factor for cardiovascular events. A cholesterol level of 6.46 mmol/l (250 mg/dl) doubles and 7.75 mmol/l (300 mg/dl) trebles the risk of cardiac death compared to 5.17 mmol/l (200 mg/dl) in postmenopausal women. The evidence for a single risk factor of hyperlipidaemia prior to the menopause increasing risk is less clear, except for women with familial hypercholesterolaemia. High-density lipoprotein (HDL) cholesterol, which is protective, is typically higher in women; therefore, it is important to get a full profile. HDL levels are inversely predictive of CHD. Hypertriglyceridaemia is a more potent risk factor for women, with the CHD relative risk increased to 32% in men and 76% in women.

The relation between lipids and stroke is complex. A meta-analysis of 61 prospective observational studies comprising almost 900,000 adults aged

40–89 years found that total cholesterol was weakly positively related to ischaemic and total stroke mortality in early middle age (40–59 years), but this finding could be largely or wholly accounted for by the association of cholesterol with blood pressure. Moreover, a positive relation was seen only in middle age and only in those with below-average blood pressure; at older ages (70–89 years) and, particularly, for those with systolic blood pressure over about 145 mmHg, total cholesterol was negatively related to haemorrhagic and total stroke mortality. Nevertheless, randomized trials show that statins substantially reduce not only coronary event rates but also total stroke rates in patients with a wide range of ages and blood pressures. Although some of the reduction in the rate of stroke may be the result of alterations in lipid levels, statins may also act through mechanisms unrelated to their lipid-lowering properties, such as improved endothelial function; plaque stabilization; and antithrombotic, anti-inflammatory and neuroprotective properties.

Diabetes

The prevalence of diabetes is increasing, and this is further compounded by the increase in obesity. In the UK, diabetes is more common in women (17.7%) than men (13.4%), and the prevalence increases in some ethnic groups, particularly Asians. The risk of CHD is increased fourfold in women and 2.5-fold in men. A woman with diabetes has a similar CHD risk to a woman who has suffered a myocardial infarct but is not diabetic. Diabetes is therefore considered to be a 'cardiovascular equivalent', and aggressive risk reduction is advocated as if a coronary event has already occurred.

Body weight, abdominal obesity and lifestyle

Increasing body weight and obesity increase the risk of CVD. These areas are covered in more detail in the sections on obesity and metabolic syndrome (see below). Lifestyle factors such as diet and exercise are discussed in Chapter 10.

Polycystic ovary syndrome

Anatomic evidence of early coronary and other vascular disease, as well as impaired endothelial function, has been found in women with polycystic ovary syndrome (PCOS). However, no prospective studies have been conducted to examine the incidence of cardiovascular events and cardiovascular mortality in women with PCOS. The lack of data is partly because most studies are conducted at a time when the individuals are young, before an age when CVD would be expected to develop. However, epidemiological data from the Women's Health Study and the Nurses' Health Study suggest that increased free androgen index and irregular menstrual cycles are associated with increased risk of CVD. Further data are awaited.

Obesity

Obesity is increasing dramatically and there is now said to be an 'epidemic'. Globally, at least one billion adults are overweight (BMI > 25), with about 300 million considered obese (BMI ≥ 30). In the USA, over 40% of adult women are obese.

The Nurses' Health Study reported in 1995 a J-shaped relation between BMI and overall mortality. In non-smokers, the relative risk (RR) of death from all causes for increasing categories of BMI were as follows: BMI < 19.0 (the reference category), RR = 1.0; 19.0–21.9, RR = 1.2; 22.0–24.9, RR = 1.2; 25.0–26.9, RR = 1.3; 27.0–28.9, RR = 1.6; 29.0–31.9, RR = 2.1; and ≥32.0, RR = 2.2 (*P* for trend <0.001). Among women with BMI of ≥32.0 who had never smoked, the RR of death from CVD was 4.1 (95% confidence interval [CI], 2.1–7.7), and that of death from cancer was 2.1 (95% CI, 1.4–3.2), as compared with the risk among women with BMI below 19.0. A weight gain of 10 kg (22 lb) or more since the age of 18 was associated with increased mortality in middle adulthood.

Obesity increases the risk of multiple health conditions such as CVD, venous thromboembolism, type 2 diabetes, cancer (endometrial, gallbladder, oesophageal adenocarcinoma, renal, breast), osteoarthritis (in both weight and non-weight bearing joints), respiratory problems and gallbladder disease. Fat distribution seems to be important. In the Nurses' Health Study, abdominal obesity is associated with increased all-cause, CVD and cancer mortality, even in normal-weight women. In reducing the ability to exercise and lose weight, obesity impairs mobility, increases the risk of falls and reduces quality of life. Furthermore, extremely obese elderly women need home care several years earlier than their normal-weight counterparts.

Metabolic syndrome

The metabolic syndrome is a combination of risk factors, including abdominal obesity, dyslipidaemia (elevated triglycerides, decreased HDL cholesterol), glucose intolerance and hypertension. It increases the risk of CVD and type 2 diabetes. The increased risk of CVD is higher in women than in men. It has been suggested that there is a metabolic syndrome resulting from the menopause due to oestrogen deficiency, as many of the risk factors are more prevalent in postmenopausal women.

Different diagnostic criteria of the metabolic syndrome have been put forward, and there is a lack of consensus on which components are fundamentally necessary and most clinically relevant. However, all the criteria include a measure of central obesity, glucose level, dyslipidaemia and hypertension, and the thresholds for some of the components vary by gender and ethnic group.

Osteoporosis

Osteoporosis is mainly a disease of older women, affecting one in three women compared to one in 12 men. Osteoporosis is defined in a National Institute of Health Consensus Statement as 'a skeletal disorder characterized by compromised bone strength predisposing to an increased risk of fracture'. Bone strength reflects the integration of two main features: bone density and bone quality. Bone density is expressed as grams of mineral per area or volume, and, in any given individual, is determined by peak bone mass and amount of bone loss. Bone quality refers to architecture, turnover, damage accumulation (for example, microfractures) and mineralization. A fracture occurs when a failure-inducing force, which may or may not involve trauma, is applied to osteoporotic bone. Thus, osteoporosis is a significant risk factor for fracture, and a distinction between risk factors that affect bone metabolism and risk factors for fracture must be made (Figure 3.1). Fractures of the wrist, hip and vertebrae, which are the main clinical manifestations of osteoporosis, have enormous impact on quality of life, result in significant economic burden, and, particularly in the case of hip fractures, are associated with considerable excess mortality. The number of hip fractures worldwide due to osteoporosis is expected to rise threefold by the middle of the century, from 1.7 million in 1990 to 6.3 million by 2050.

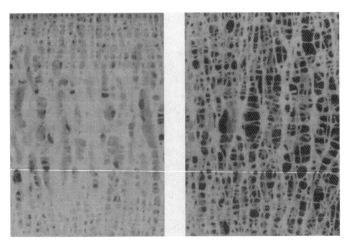

Figure 3.1 Normal (left) and osteoporotic bone (right)

Clinical consequences of osteoporosis

Fractures are the clinical consequences of osteoporosis. By the age of 80 years, most women will have sustained one or more fractures of varying severity. The most common sites of osteoporotic fractures are as follows:

- lower end of radius (wrist or Colles' fracture)
- proximal femur (hip)
- vertebrae.

Other sites include pelvis, ribs, humerus and distal femur. Fractures have a major impact on quality of life, result in a significant economic burden and, particularly in the case of hip fractures, are associated with considerable excess mortality.

Colles' fractures frequently occur after a fall onto an outstretched hand. Although such fractures seldom require hospitalization, they are very painful and considerably reduce mobility and function.

Hip fracture in young patients is usually the result of traffic accidents. In older patients, however, hip fractures are caused by falls or may even occur spontaneously. The incidence of hip fracture is about twice as high in women as in men. In many Western countries, the remaining lifetime risk of a hip fracture in Caucasian women at the age of menopause is about 14%. Hip fracture is associated with more deaths, disability and medical costs than all other osteoporotic fractures combined. In the year after a hip fracture, mortality is about 30%. Some 50% of patients who survive hip fractures have permanent disability and fail to regain their previous level of independence.

Vertebral fractures are difficult to quantify, as many patients remain asymptomatic until considerable deformity has occurred. Vertebral fractures often present as non-specific back pain and may be undiagnosed for many years. Indeed, as many as nine of 10 of such fractures are estimated never to come under medical attention. Vertebral fractures lead to a loss of height and curvature of the spine, with the typical dorsal kyphosis ('dowager's hump'). Multiple fractures may give rise to loss of height and considerable loss of quality of life, and ultimately may impair respiratory function. Even one vertebral fracture is a powerful predictor of future vertebral and other osteoporotic fractures. The prevention of the first fracture and the identification of individuals at risk of this is a central goal of research in osteoporosis.

The cost of osteoporotic fracture is high. Worldwide, the cost of hip fractures is estimated to be US$34,800m in 1990 and to reach US$131,500m in 2050. In the UK, the National Health Service (NHS)'s annual expenditure on the acute care and after care of osteoporosis-related fractures is close to £1.7bn. This figure does not encompass the economic costs of family members diversion from economic activity to caring.

Definitions of osteoporosis according to the World Health Organization

On the basis of the measurement of bone mineral density (BMD) (Table 3.3), the World Health Organization (WHO)'s definitions, applied to postmenopausal women, result in 30% of this population being classified as having osteoporosis. Severe osteoporosis is defined as the presence of fragility or minimal trauma fracture (fracture after a fall from a chair or standing) and low BMD (T score less than –2.5). The T score is that number of standard deviations (SD) by which the bone in question differs from the young normal mean. Although BMD is a major contributor to risk, other factors, including age, BMI, falls, bone quality and rate of bone resorption and formation, play a part in determining whether or not a person will sustain a fracture.

Determinants of bone mass

Age and gender

Bone density increases during the growth periods of the teenage years, reaching a peak sometime during the mid-20s. Peak bone density is then sustained for some years and begins to decline during the mid-40s. After the menopause, an accelerated period of bone loss occurs, which lasts for 6–10 years. Thereafter, bone loss continues but at a much slower rate (Figure 3.2). Any bone has a 'threshold' value of bone mass below which the bone will fracture after minor trauma.

Whether or not a postmenopausal woman develops osteoporosis is determined largely by her peak bone mass, rate of postmenopausal bone loss and longevity. One of the reasons men generally develop osteoporosis only late in life is because they have a much higher peak bone mass than women and do not have the accelerated decade of loss consequent on the female endocrine menopause. Intuitively, some of the measures to prevent osteoporosis would include encouragement in childhood and adolescence of a diet replete in

Table 3.3

Definitions of osteoporosis according to the World Health Organization

Description	Definition
Normal	BMD value between –1 SD and +1 SD of the young adult mean (T score –1 to +1)
Osteopenia	BMD reduced by between –1 and –2.5 SD from the young adult mean (T score –1 to –2.5)
Osteoporosis	BMD reduced by equal to or more than –2.5 SD from the young adult mean (T score –2.5 or lower)

BMD, body mass index

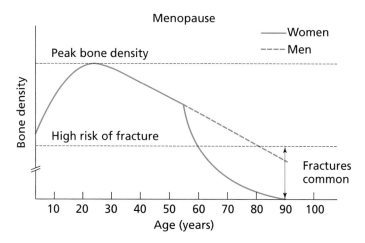

Figure 3.2 Pattern of bone mass with age

calcium and vitamin D coupled with weight-bearing exercise and discouragement of smoking in adolescence to enhance peak bone mass. Studies are required, however, to examine the efficacy of these interventions.

Ethnicity and genetic factors

An ethnic variation in the susceptibility to osteoporosis exists, with Caucasian women, for example, having a higher rate of fracture than women of African-Caribbean origin.

Twin and family studies have shown that genetic factors contribute to osteoporosis by influencing BMD and other determinants of fracture risk such as ultrasound properties of bone, skeletal geometry and bone turnover. It is unlikely, however, that a single gene defect exists for osteoporosis, but several candidates that influence BMD have been examined, including those for the vitamin D receptor, oestrogen receptor and collagen. General agreement, however, is that bone density is determined largely by genetic factors, with environmental influences playing a lesser role.

Risk factors for the development of osteoporosis

Specific populations at greatly increased risk of osteoporotic fracture can be identified (Table 3.4). Although these risk factors have been useful at a population level, their use in clinical practice to assess an individual's risk of osteoporosis is difficult, as the increased risk with some factors is small. The factors most important in clinical practice to alert the health professional to

Table 3.4

Risk factors for osteoporosis

Risk factor	Example
Genetic	Family history of fracture (particularly first-degree relative with hip fracture)
Constitutional	Low body mass index (BMI)
	Early menopause (<45 years of age)
Environmental	Cigarette smoking
	Alcohol abuse
	Low calcium intake
	Sedentary lifestyle
Drugs	Corticosteroids, >5 mg prednisolone or equivalent daily
Diseases	Rheumatoid arthritis
	Neuromuscular disease
	Chronic liver disease
	Malabsorption syndrome
	Hyperparathyroidism
	Hyperthyroidism
	Hypogonadism

the possible risk are family history of fracture (particularly a first-degree relative with hip fracture), early menopause, chronic use of corticosteroids (oral and possibly inhaled), prolonged immobilization and prior fracture.

Depot medroxyprogesterone acetate contraception

The relation between BMD and the use of depot medroxyprogesterone acetate (DMPA) is complex. The amenorrhoea induced by DMPA contraception is associated with a 5–10% loss of bone, which occurs when used before but not after when peak bone mass is achieved. It is not progressive and seems to reverse rapidly on stopping DMPA.

It would be prudent to assess the patient's risk factors for osteoporosis. Thus, a woman who has a normal BMI with a good diet and exercise pattern, is probably safe. However, if she has a family history of osteoporosis, is underweight, and has a personal history of poor diet, exercise and smoking, an estimate of bone density should be considered. If the results are in the osteopenic range, an alternative means of contraception should be discussed. In any case, DMPA should probably be discontinued at age 40 years to allow resumption of ovarian cycling for the remaining 10 years or so up to the natural menopause. The long-term skeletal effects of DMPA in teenagers who have yet to achieve peak bone mass is presently uncertain, and its use has to be balanced against the benefits of a very effective form of contraception.

Dementia and cognitive decline

'Dementia' is a clinical term used to describe a condition in which there is impairment of cognitive faculties, including loss of memory, language, thinking and judgement, causing significant difficulties in daily functioning. A wide variety of disorders can cause dementia. The most common are Alzheimer's disease, vascular dementia and dementia with Lewy bodies; frontotemporal dementia accounts for about one-tenth of cases. Mild cognitive impairment refers to cognitive difficulties exceeding those expected on the basis of normal ageing but not severe enough to represent dementia. Particularly when memory is affected, mild cognitive impairment increases the chances of a future diagnosis of Alzheimer's disease.

Worldwide, about 25 million people have dementia, with 4.6 million new cases of dementia every year (one new case every 7 s). It is estimated that the number of people affected will double every 20 years to 81.1 million by 2040. Most people with dementia live in developing countries (60% in 2001, rising to 71% by 2040). Rates of increase are not uniform; numbers in developed countries are forecast to increase by 100% between 2001 and 2040, but by more than 300% in India, China, and their south Asian and western Pacific neighbours. In the UK, there are an estimated 750,000 people with dementia, and this includes over 18,000 people aged under 65 years. In the USA, there are 4–5 million sufferers.

Dementia is a common but not inevitable consequence of ageing. Its prevalence and incidence increase with age, and the risk of developing dementia doubles every 5 years after age 65. Only about 1–2% of people aged 65 years are affected, increasing to at least 20% in people aged 80 years and over. It may exceed 50% in those over 90.

The average life expectancy of a person with dementia is 3–7 years after the diagnosis is made, although diagnosis often occurs some years after first onset of symptoms. Dementia causes significant distress to patients and their carers and families, and has an enormous impact on society. Most people with dementia live in the community and require a range of supportive services, and in the long term they are likely to require residential or nursing home care. Indeed, an estimated 50% of all nursing home residents suffer from dementia. Women have a central role in providing care and support to people with dementia, either as a member of a family or as a voluntary or aid carer.

Respiratory problems: chronic obstructive pulmonary disease and asthma

Chronic obstructive pulmonary disease (COPD) is a lung disease characterized by chronic obstruction of lung airflow that interferes with normal breathing and is not fully reversible. The more familiar terms 'chronic bronchitis' and 'emphysema' are no longer used, but are now included within the COPD diagnosis. The primary cause of COPD is tobacco smoke (including second-hand or passive exposure). Other risk factors include:

- indoor air pollution (such as biomass fuel used for cooking and heating)
- outdoor air pollution
- occupational dusts and chemicals (vapours, irritants and fumes)
- frequent lower respiratory infections during childhood.

According to the WHO, 210 million people currently have COPD, and 3 million people, of whom 1.4 million were women, died of COPD in 2005, corresponding to 5% of all deaths globally. WHO predicts that COPD will become the fourth leading cause of death worldwide by 2030. At one time, COPD was more common in men, but because of increased tobacco use among women in high-income countries and the higher risk of exposure to indoor air pollution (such as biomass fuel used for cooking and heating) in low-income countries, the disease now affects men and women almost equally. About 250 million women worldwide smoke.

Asthma is a chronic disease characterized by recurrent attacks of breathlessness and wheezing, which vary in severity and frequency from person to person. Symptoms may occur several times in a day or week in affected individuals, and, for some people, become worse during physical activity or at night. According to the WHO, 300 million people suffer from asthma and 255,000 people died of asthma in 2005.

Management of both conditions may involve the use of corticosteroids, either systemic or inhaled, which may adversely affect the skeleton.

Urogenital atrophy and urinary incontinence

The lower urinary and genital tracts have a common embryological origin and are approximated closely in adult women. Oestrogen receptors and progesterone receptors are present in the vagina, urethra, bladder and pelvic floor musculature. In urogenital atrophy, the vaginal epithelium becomes thin and loses its rugae and becomes pale or erythematous with fine petechial haemorrhages. The maturation index shifts, leading to basal and parabasal cells in the surface layer. An increase in vaginal pH, due to lower production of lactic acid, permits the growth of pathogens. Vaginal and cervical secretions also decrease, leading to reduced lubrication. The resulting symptoms include dyspareunia, itching, burning and dryness, which can coexist with urinary symptoms (Table 3.5). Urogenital atrophy is common, affecting about 25% of women even if they are taking systemic oestrogen replacement.

Table 3.5

Symptoms of urogenital atrophy

Site of atrophy	Symptoms
Vaginal	• Vaginal dryness • Vaginal burning • Pruritus • Dyspareunia • Prolapse
Urinary	• Urgency • Frequency • Dysuria • Urinary tract infection • Incontinence • Voiding difficulties

Urinary incontinence (UI) affects millions of women throughout the world (Box 3.1). It affects the quality of life of women of all ages and poses a large financial burden on society. The EPINCONT Norwegian study found that 25% of women aged 20 to over 90 years reported involuntary loss of urine. The prevalence of UI rose with increasing age. The lowest prevalence was observed in the younger age groups (12% for women under 30 years), the highest was observed among the eldest (40% for women over 90 years). However, there was also a peak around middle age, with a prevalence of 30% among women aged 50–54 years. In the USA, the population-based prevalence of UI has been estimated to be 45%. Prevalence increased with age, from 28% for 30–39-year-old women to 55% for 80–90-year-old women.

Box 3.1

Definitions of incontinence

Urinary incontinence: the complaint of any involuntary leakage of urine
Stress urinary incontinence: involuntary leakage triggered by physical exertion, sneezing or coughing
Urge urinary incontinence: involuntary leakage accompanied by or immediately preceded by urgency
Mixed urinary incontinence: involuntary leakage associated with urgency and also with physical exertion, sneezing or coughing
Nocturnal enuresis: loss of urine occurring during sleep
Continuous urinary incontinence: complaint of continuous leakage
Coital incontinence: involuntary leakage during sexual intercourse

Other causes of incontinence include urinary fistulae, diverticulae, functional incontinence, or psychogenic causes

Adapted from Abrams *et al* 2002

Eighteen percent of respondents reported severe UI. The prevalence of severe UI also increased notably with age, from 8% for 30–39-year-old women to 33% for 80–90-year-old women. Other surveys have produced similar results. Although urogenital atrophy and UI are common, numbers seeking medical help are low, suggesting that women are suffering in silence.

Further reading

General references

Mathers CD, Loncar D. Projections of global mortality and burden of disease from 2002 to 2030. *PLoS Med* 2006;**3**:e442.

Michel JP, Newton JL, Kirkwood TB. Medical challenges of improving the quality of a longer life. *JAMA* 2008;**299**:688–90.

Ribeiro PS, Jacobsen KH, Mathers CD, Garcia-Moreno C. Priorities for women's health from the Global Burden of Disease study. *Int J Gynaecol Obstet* 2008;**102**: 82–90.

Cardiovascular disease

Allender S, Scarborough P, Peto V, *et al.* European cardiovascular disease statistics 2008. European Heart Network. www.heartstats.org/datapage.asp?id =7683.

Bello N, Mosca L. Epidemiology of coronary heart disease in women. *Prog Cardiovasc Dis* 2004;**46**:287–95.

Bolego C, Poli A, Paoletti R. Smoking and gender. *Cardiovasc Res* 2002;**53**:568–76.

British Heart Foundation. www.heartstats.org.

Bushnell CD. Stroke and the female brain. *Nat Clin Pract Neurol* 2008;**4**:22–33.

Centers for Disease Control and Prevention United States. Leading causes of death in females, 2004. www.cdc.gov/women/lcod.htm.

Collins P, Rosano G, Casey C, *et al.* Management of cardiovascular risk in the perimenopausal woman: a consensus statement of European cardiologists and gynaecologists. *Eur Heart J* 2007;**28**:2028–40.

Conroy RM, Pyörälä K, Fitzgerald AP, *et al.*; SCORE project group. Estimation of ten-year risk of fatal cardiovascular disease in Europe: the SCORE project. *Eur Heart J* 2003;**24**:987–1003.

Ford ES, Ajani UA, Croft JB, *et al.* Explaining the decrease in US deaths from coronary disease, 1980–2000. *N Engl J Med* 2007;**356**:2388–98.

Hoffman LK, Ehrmann DA. Cardiometabolic features of polycystic ovary syndrome. *Nat Clin Pract Endocrinol Metab* 2008;**4**:215–22.

Jackson G. Gender differences in cardiovascular disease prevention. *Menopause Int* 2008;**14**:13–17.

JBS 2: Joint British Societies guidelines on prevention of cardiovascular disease in clinical practice. *Heart* 2005;**91**(Suppl 5):1–52.

LaRosa JC, Hunninghake D, Bush D, *et al.* The cholesterol facts. A summary of the evidence relating dietary fats, serum cholesterol, and coronary heart disease. A joint statement by the American Heart Association and the National Heart, Lung and Blood Institute. Task Force on Cholesterol Issues, American Heart Association. *Circulation* 1990;**81**:1721–33.

Mosca L, Banka CL, Benjamin EJ, *et al.* Evidence-based guidelines for cardiovascular disease prevention in women: 2007 update. *J Am Coll Cardiol* 2007;**49**:1230–50.

National Heart, Lung and Blood Institute. 2007 NHLBI Morbidity and Mortality Chart Book. www.nhlbi.nih.gov/resources.

Nissen SE, Tuzcu EM, Libby P, *et al.* Effect of antihypertensive agents on cardiovascular events in patients with coronary disease and normal blood pressure. The CAMELOT Study: a randomised controlled trial. *JAMA* 2004;**292**:2217–26.

Prospective Studies Collaboration; Lewington S, Whitlock G, Clarke R, *et al.* Blood cholesterol and vascular mortality by age, sex, and blood pressure: a meta-analysis of individual data from 61 prospective studies with 55,000 vascular deaths. *Lancet* 2007;**370**:1829–39.

Rosamond W, Flegal K, Friday G, *et al.* Epidemiology of coronary heart disease in women. *Heart* 2006;**92**(Suppl 3):iii2–iii4.

Stramba-Badiale M, Fox KM, Priori SG, *et al.* Cardiovascular disease in women: a statement from the policy conference of the European Society of Cardiology. *Eur Heart J* 2006;**27**:994–1005.

Wasserthiel-Smoller S, Hong Y; American Heart Association Statistics Committee and Stroke Statistics Subcommittee. Heart disease and stroke statistics – 2007 update: a report from the American Heart Association Statistics Committee and Stroke Statistics Subcommittee. *Circulation* 2007;**115**:e69–171.

Williams B. Recent hypertension trials: implications and controversies. *J Am Coll Cardiol* 2005;**45**:814–27.

Obesity and metabolic syndrome

Alberti KG, Zimmet P, Shaw J; IDF Epidemiology Task Force Consensus Group. The metabolic syndrome: a new worldwide definition. *Lancet* 2005;**366**:1059–62.

Balkau B, Charles MA. Comment on the provisional report from the WHO consultation. European Group for the Study of Insulin Resistance (EGIR). *Diabet Med* 1999;**16**:442–3.

Einhorn D, Reaven GM, Cobin RH, *et al.* American College of Endocrinology position statement on the insulin resistance syndrome. *Endocr Pract* 2003;**9**:237–52.

Fjeldstad C, Fjeldstad AS, Acree LS, *et al.* The influence of obesity on falls and quality of life. *Dyn Med* 2008;**7**:4.

Galassi A, Reynolds K, He J. Metabolic syndrome and risk of cardiovascular disease: a meta-analysis. *Am J Med* 2006;**119**:812–19.

Grundy SM, Cleeman JI, Daniels SR, *et al.* American Heart Association; National Heart, Lung, and Blood Institute. Diagnosis and management of the metabolic syndrome: an American Heart Association/National Heart, Lung, and Blood Institute Scientific Statement. *Circulation* 2005;**112**:2735–52.

Kaaja RJ. Metabolic syndrome and the menopause. *Menopause Int* 2008;**14**:21–5.

Liu B, Balkwill A, Banks E, *et al.* Relationship of height, weight and body mass index to the risk of hip and knee replacements in middle-aged women. *Rheumatology (Oxford)* 2007;**46**:861–7.

Magliano M. Obesity and arthritis. *Menopause Int* 2008;**14**:149–54.

Manson JE, Willett WC, Stampfer MJ, *et al.* Body weight and mortality among women. *N Engl J Med* 1995;**333**:677–85.

National Cholesterol Education Program. Executive Summary of the Third Report of the National Cholesterol Education Program (NCEP) Expert Panel on Detection, Evaluation, and Treatment of High Blood Cholesterol in Adults (Adult Treatment Panel III). *JAMA* 2001;**285**:2486–97.

Patterson RE, Frank LL, Kristal AR, White E. A comprehensive examination of health conditions associated with obesity in older adults. *Am J Prev Med* 2004;**27**:385–90.

Reeves GK, Pirie K, Beral V, *et al.*; Million Women Study Collaboration. Cancer incidence and mortality in relation to body mass index in the Million Women Study: cohort study. *BMJ* 2007;**335**:1107–8.

Renehan AG, Tyson M, Egger M, *et al.* Body-mass index and incidence of cancer: a systematic review and meta-analysis of prospective observational studies. *Lancet* 2008;**371**:569–78.

Sørbye LW, Schroll M, Finne-Soveri H, *et al.*; AdHOC Project Research Group. Home care needs of extremely obese elderly European women. *Menopause Int* 2007;**13**:84–7.

Spencer CP, Godsland IF, Stevenson JC. Is there a menopausal metabolic syndrome? *Gynecol Endocrinol* 1997;**11**:341–55.

World Health Organization. WHO Global Infobase Online, Country Comparable Data. www.who.int/infobase/report.aspx.

Zhang C, Rexrode KM, van Dam RM, *et al.* Abdominal obesity and the risk of all-cause, cardiovascular, and cancer mortality: sixteen years of follow-up in US women. *Circulation* 2008;**117**:1658–67.

Osteoporosis

Clark MK, Sowers M, Levy B, Nichols S. Bone mineral density loss and recovery during 48 months in first-time users of depot medroxyprogesterone acetate. *Fertil Steril* 2006;**86**:1466–74.

Johnell O. The socioeconomic burden of fractures: today and in the 21st century. *Am J Med* 1997;**103**:S20–5.

Johnell O, Kanis J. Epidemiology of osteoporotic fractures. *Osteoporos Int* 2005;**16**(Suppl 2):S3–7.

NIH Consensus Development Panel on Osteoporosis Prevention, Diagnosis, and Therapy. Osteoporosis prevention, diagnosis, and therapy. *JAMA* 2001;**285**: 785–95.

Poole KES, Compston JE. Osteoporosis and its management. *BMJ* 2006;**333**:1251–6.

Ralston SH. Genetics of osteoporosis. *Proc Nutr Soc* 2007;**66**:158–65.

Scholes D, LaCroix AZ, Ichikawa LE, *et al.* Change in bone mineral density among adolescent women using and discontinuing depot medroxyprogesterone acetate contraception. *Arch Pediatr Adolesc Med* 2005;**159**:139–44.

Walsh JS, Eastell R, Peel NF. Effects of depot medroxyprogesterone acetate on bone density and bone metabolism before and after peak bone mass: a case-control study. *J Clin Endocrinol Metab* 2008;**93**:1317–23.

World Health Organization. Assessment of fracture risk and its application to screening for postmenopausal osteoporosis. WHO Technical Report Series 843. Geneva: WHO, 1994.

Dementia and cognitive decline

Alzheimer's Society. www.alzheimers.org.uk/site/index.php.

Chapman DP, Williams SM, Strine TW, *et al*. Dementia and its implications for public health. *Prev Chronic Dis* 2006;**3**:A34.

Ferri CP, Prince M, Brayne C, *et al.*; Alzheimer's Disease International. Global prevalence of dementia: a Delphi consensus study. *Lancet* 2005;**366**:2112–17.

Gauthier S, Reisberg B, Zaudig M, *et al*. Mild cognitive impairment. *Lancet* 2006;**21**: 1262–70.

Thomas AJ, O'Brien JT. Depression and cognition in older adults. *Curr Opin Psychiatry* 2008;**21**:8–13.

Respiratory problems

Quon BS, Gan WQ, Sin DD. Contemporary management of acute exacerbations of COPD: a systematic review and metaanalysis. *Chest* 2008;**133**:756–66.

Sin DD, Man J, Sharpe H, *et al*. Pharmacological management to reduce exacerbations in adults with asthma: a systematic review and meta-analysis. *JAMA* 2004;**292**: 367–76.

World Health Organization. Chronic obstructive pulmonary disease (COPD). www.who.int/mediacentre/factsheets/fs315/en/index.html.

World Health Organization. Asthma. www.who.int/mediacentre/factsheets/fs307/en/index.html.

Urogenital atrophy and urinary incontinence

Abrams P, Cardozo L, Fall M, *et al*. The standardization of terminology of lower urinary tract function: report from the standardization subcommittee of the International Continence Society. *Neurourol Urodyn* 2002;**21**:167–78.

American College of Obstetricians and Gynecologists Women's Health Care Physicians. Genitourinary tract changes. *Obstet Gynecol* 2004;**104**(Suppl 4): S56–61.

Castelo-Branco C, Cancelo MJ, Villero J, *et al*. Management of post-menopausal vaginal atrophy and atrophic vaginitis. *Maturitas* 2005;**52**(Suppl 1):S46–52.

Hannestad YS, Rortveit G, Hunskaar S. Help-seeking and associated factors in female urinary incontinence. The Norwegian EPINCONT Study. Epidemiology of Incontinence in the County of Nord-Trøndelag. *Scand J Prim Health Care* 2002;**20**:102–7.

Hannestad YS, Rortveit G, Sandvik H, Hunskaar S; Norwegian EPINCONT study. Epidemiology of Incontinence in the County of Nord-Trøndelag. A community-based epidemiological survey of female urinary incontinence: the Norwegian

EPINCONT study. Epidemiology of Incontinence in the County of Nord-Trondelag. *J Clin Epidemiol* 2000;**53**:1150–7.

Hunskaar S, Lose G, Sykes D, Voss S. The prevalence of urinary incontinence in women in four European countries. *BJU Int* 2004;**93**:324–30.

Melville JL, Katon W, Delaney K, Newton K. Urinary incontinence in US women: a population-based study. *Arch Intern Med* 2005;**165**:537–42.

Minassian VA, Stewart WF, Wood GC. Urinary incontinence in women: variation in prevalence estimates and risk factors. *Obstet Gynecol* 2008;**111**(2 Pt 1):324–31.

Shaw C, Gupta RD, Bushnell DM, *et al*. The extent and severity of urinary incontinence amongst women in UK GP waiting rooms. *Fam Pract* 2006;**23**:497–506.

ASSESSMENT AND INVESTIGATIONS

4 Initial assessment, follow-up and contraception

> Assessment
> Examination and screening
> Follow-up
> Contraception
> Further reading

Consultations about the menopause are becoming more complex because of the wide range of therapeutic options, the controversies regarding hormone replacement therapy (HRT), and the increasing use of alternative and complementary therapies. This chapter describes assessment, follow-up and contraception.

Assessment

The following discussion details useful information that can be obtained from the patient and underpins any further assessment. It is important to ascertain menopausal status and risk factors for cardiovascular disease and osteoporosis, as well as the woman's personal views on the menopause itself and on any interventions (Box 4.1).

Examination and screening

Physical examination should include recording of body mass index (BMI) and blood pressure. Whether breast or pelvic examination should be undertaken initially and then at regular intervals is a controversial area, with practice varying worldwide. In the UK, regulatory bodies advise that clinical examination of the breasts and pelvic examination are not *routinely* necessary in all HRT users, but they must be performed if clinically indicated. The words 'clinically indicated' for pelvic examination should relate to past or current disease, symptoms or family history. It is important not to miss a breast or a pelvic mass or a pregnancy.

Women should also be encouraged to participate in national screening programmes for cervical and breast cancer. In the UK, the cervical screening

Box 4.1

Patient assessment

Symptoms, menstrual history and contraception
- Hot flushes and night sweats
- Vaginal dryness
- Sexual problems
- Other symptoms
- Date of last menstrual period (could she be pregnant?)
- Frequency, heaviness and duration of periods
- Contraception

Personal or family medical problems
1. Breast, ovarian or bowel cancer in close family members
   - Have any parents, sisters or brothers or the patient had such cancers?
   - If so, at what age did they develop it?
2. Deep vein thrombosis or pulmonary embolism
   - Have any parents, brothers or sisters or the patient had such conditions?
   - If so, when and why did this happen?
     - Was it after a hip or knee replacement?
     - Was the person on the 'pill' or pregnant?
   - Did they have any test to confirm the clot?
   - Was the clinical suspicion confirmed?
   - Were they treated with anticoagulants such as heparin or warfarin?
3. Risk factors for heart disease and strokes
   - Has the patient already had a heart attack or stroke?
   - Have her parents, brothers or sisters had a myocardial infarction or stroke, and, if so, at what age?
   - Does the patient smoke, and, if so, how many cigarettes a day?
   - Does the patient have hypertension or diabetes?
   - Does the patient have a high cholesterol level?
4. Risk factors for osteoporosis
   - Was the menopause before the age of 45 years?
   - Has the patient taken systemic corticosteroids for 6 months or longer?
   - Has the patient had anorexia or significant weight loss?
   - Does the patient have a family history of osteoporosis (especially in her mother or sister)?
   - Has the patient had low calcium or vitamin D intake or deficiency, or malabsorption disorders?
   - Has the patient already had a fracture? If so, was it from standing height, how did it happen and where was it?
5. Other
   - Has the patient had migraine?
   - What medicines are being taken, including herbal remedies and vitamin supplements?
   - Is the patient at risk of pregnancy?
6. What does the patient want?
   - Does she want to take HRT?
   - If yes, what preparation would she prefer – and by what route?
   - If not, what are her most important treatment endpoints?

It is a woman's evidence-based patient choice to take or not to take HRT or any therapy, and her decision must be recorded in the notes.

programme, invites women aged 25–64 years for screening. The frequency of mammography screening programmes varies between countries and is about every 2–3 years. In the UK, the mammography screening programme invites all women aged 50–70 for mammography every 3 years and is available on request to women older than 70 years. There is no need for additional mammography or cervical screening in HRT users.

Follow-up

After instigating a particular type of treatment, the patient should be seen for follow-up after about 3 months. This is because most symptoms will have responded to oestrogen- or non-oestrogen-based treatments by this time. In addition, persistence of any side-effects will be apparent. At 3 months, the practitioner can decide on the management of residual difficulties. Controversy surrounds the frequency of follow-up thereafter. In the UK, the Medicines and Healthcare Products Regulatory Agency recommends that HRT 'be re-evaluated at least annually in light of new knowledge and any changes in a woman's risk factors'. It is probably prudent to arrange annual follow-up for any treatment (both oestrogen- and non-oestrogen-based), as the risks and benefits of any particular strategy for each individual woman will alter with time and need to be discussed. The need for oestrogen often declines with age.

Monitoring of blood pressure is not needed routinely in HRT users. Studies of the effects of natural oestrogens have found slight increases and decreases in blood pressure. In general, blood pressure does not change. Rarely, conjugated equine oestrogens cause severe hypertension, but this returns to normal when treatment is stopped. In patients whose pre-existing hypertension has been treated to normalize or reduce blood pressure, oestrogens can be given safely (see Chapter 14). Blood pressure should be monitored regularly at 6-month intervals, as would be good clinical practice in any hypertensive patient. Postmenopausal bleeding and any abnormal bleeding, whether women are taking HRT or not, should always be investigated. It is essential to investigate for cervical or endometrial cancer.

Contraception

Perimenopausal women cannot be assumed to be infertile, and there are well-documented records of births to women in their 50s. The oldest woman known to have given birth after a spontaneous conception was aged 57 years and 129 days. When an unplanned pregnancy occurs, it can be a disaster and both abortion and childbirth are associated with a higher morbidity and mortality. Older women have a higher risk of pregnancy-induced hypertension, pre-eclampsia and gestational diabetes. The risk of fetal malformation increases, with an increase in chromosomal disorders such as Down's syndrome, as does the risk of miscarriage. Contraceptive options thus must be considered carefully.

Duration of contraceptive use in the perimenopause

The normal recommendation is to continue contraception after the final menstrual period for at least 2 years if the woman is younger than 50 years and at least one year if she is older than 50. Condoms can continue to be used in postmenopausal women to reduce the risk of transmission of sexually transmitted diseases.

The final menstrual period can be identified only retrospectively and may be difficult to identify in women who use a contraceptive method that renders them amenorrhoeic and in those who take a combined oral contraceptive or monthly sequential HRT that induces cyclical withdrawal bleeding. Elevated levels of follicle-stimulating hormone (FSH) after stopping oral contraceptives or HRT do not reliably indicate infertility. Hormone replacement therapy does not provide contraception.

Contraceptive options in the perimenopause

A variety of contraceptive methods are available, and their suitability for perimenopausal women is detailed in Box 4.2.

Box 4.2

Contraceptive options for perimenopausal women

Natural family planning
- Unpredictable cycles, inconsistent temperature changes and atypical mucous changes in the perimenopause make the method unreliable.
- Methods that depend on the detection of the hormonal changes at ovulation are unreliable.

Coitus interruptus
- Unreliable but a method of choice for some couples.
- Vaginal dryness, fear of pregnancy and concomitant changes in libido and potency may alter acceptability.

Condoms
- Ongoing use is acceptable but may cause discomfort.
- Risk of rupture is increased in association with mucosal atrophic changes.
- Lubricating or spermicidal gels should be recommended.

Diaphragm
- Continued use is acceptable.
- Mucosal atrophy or prolapse of the vaginal wall, or both, may cause difficulties with fitting or retention.

Spermicides
- May help lubrication, and efficacy increases with age.
- Should be used with barrier methods or as a single method, such as foam.
- Vaginal atrophic changes can lead to increased sensitivity with mucosal inflammation and breakdown.

Intrauterine devices
- Ongoing use is appropriate if already *in situ* at the time of the menopause, and they may be left in for more than 5 years until contraception is no longer required.
- May increase the incidence of abnormal bleeding.

Intrauterine systems
- Intrauterine devices that contain progestogen suppress the endometrium, leading to amenorrhoea in many women, and can be used to treat menorrhagia.
- May be used with systemic oestrogen and provide 'period-free' HRT in the perimenopause.

Combined contraception (oral, patch and vaginal ring)
- Low-dose, combined contraceptives provide reliable contraception, as well as benefits of oestrogen replacement in older women.
- Non-smokers and normotensive, non-obese women can continue low-dose combined pills until at least their mid-40s or early 50s.
- May potentiate the age-related increase in cardiovascular and cerebrovascular disease.
- Risk of breast cancer may be slightly increased.

Progestogen-only pills
- Are suitable for use throughout the perimenopause, with no upper age limit for their use.
- Efficacy improves with age.
- Use in combination with systemic HRT has not been well evaluated.

Intramuscular progestogens and subdermal progestogens
- Amenorrhoea makes it difficult to identify the menopause.
- Use in combination with systemic HRT has not been well evaluated.
- Potential adverse effects of intramuscular progestogens, such as depot Provera, on bone mass may limit their use.

Sterilization (male or female)
- This is the most common form of pregnancy prevention in perimenopausal women in some countries such as the UK.

Note: Some vaginal preparations, including oestrogen creams and pessaries and non-hormonal lubricants, may damage the rubber used in condoms and diaphragms, leading to increased risk of rupture

Further reading

American College of Obstetricians and Gynecologists. ACOG Practice Bulletin no. 45. Cervical cytology screening. *Obstet Gynecol* 2003;**102**:417–27.

American College of Physicians PIER, Physicians Information and Education Resource, Menopause and Hormone Therapy. pier.acponline.org.

Confidential Enquiry into Maternal and Child Health. Saving Mothers' Lives 2003–2005. London: CEMACH Publications, 2007.

Faculty of Family Planning and Reproductive Health Care Clinical Effectiveness Unit. Contraception for women aged over 40 years. *J Fam Plann Reprod Health Care* 2005;**31**:51–64.

Gebbie A. Contraception in the perimenopause. In: Tomlinson JM, Rees M, Mander A, eds. *Sexual Health and the Menopause*. London: RSM Press, 2005:47–54.

Kösters JP, Gøtzsche PC. Regular self-examination or clinical examination for early detection of breast cancer. *Cochrane Database Syst Rev* 2008;**3**:CD003373.

NHS Breast Screening Programme. www.cancerscreening.nhs.uk/breastscreen.

Practice Committee of the American Society for Reproductive Medicine. Hormonal contraception: recent advances and controversies. *Fertil Steril* 2006;**86**(5 Suppl): S229–35.

5 Investigations and screening

Endocrine investigations
Skeletal assessment
Risk factors for cardiovascular disease
Mammography and genetic testing
Endometrial assessment
Further reading

Endocrine investigations

Gonadotrophins and ovarian steroids

Levels of follicle-stimulating hormone (FSH) are helpful only if the diagnosis of climacteric symptoms is in doubt and the levels are reported in the menopausal range (>30 IU/l). In the perimenopause, the daily variation in levels of FSH renders this parameter of limited value (see Chapter 1). Levels of FSH do not predict when the last menstrual period will occur and are not a guide to fertility status, as increased levels can occur in the presence of ovulatory cycles. They are also of little value in monitoring hormone replacement therapy (HRT), as this gonadotrophin is controlled by inhibin as well as oestradiol in normal physiology. Furthermore, FSH levels decline and with increasing age can be in the premenopausal range in women over 60. It needs to be measured, however, in women with suspected premature ovarian failure, whether or not they are hysterectomized. The blood sample is best collected on days 3–5 of the cycle (day 1 is the first day of menstruation). Where this is not possible – as in women with oligomenorrhoea or amenorrhoea, or women who have undergone hysterectomy – two samples separated by an interval of 2 weeks should be obtained.

Estimates of the levels of luteinizing hormone (LH), oestradiol, progesterone and testosterone are of no value in the diagnosis of ovarian failure. Levels of oestradiol may be of some value in checking absorption of oestradiol delivered by the non-oral route. They should not be used, however, when oestrogen is given orally, as the major circulating metabolite in this case is oestrone.

Thyroid function tests (free thyroxine [T4] and thyroid-stimulating hormone)

Abnormalities of thyroid function (which lead to lethargy, weight gain, hair loss and flushes) often can be confused with menopausal symptoms, and thyroid function tests should be done whenever the signs and symptoms are appropriate, particularly if the patient has an inadequate symptomatic response to HRT.

Catecholamines and 5-hydroxyindolacetic acid

Levels of catecholamines in the urine over 24 hours are used in the diagnosis of phaeochromocytoma – a rare cause of hot flushes. Levels of 5-hydroxyin-dolacetic acid in urine over 24 hours are used in the diagnosis of carcinoid syndrome – another rare cause of hot flushes.

Testosterone levels

Women who complain of lack of libido may request measurement of levels of testosterone. In women, however, slightly more than two-thirds of circulating testosterone is bound to steroid hormone binding globulin (SHBG), and a further one-third is weakly bound to albumin, leaving around 2% of the total testosterone in the free or unbound state. As concentrations of SHBG can fluctuate, total levels of testosterone do not yield meaningful information about exposure of the tissues to androgens. A free testosterone index accurately evaluates the tissue androgen status but is not available routinely in clinical practice. Low circulating levels of androgens have been proposed to be associated with low sexual desire; however, no level of a single androgen is predictive of low sexual function in women.

Skeletal assessment

General agreement is that population screening for osteoporosis is not advised. Much can be gained, however, by the selective examination of women from groups at particular risk (Figure 5.1).

Dual energy X-ray absorptiometry

Dual energy X-ray absorptiometry (DXA) is an X-ray-based system that uses two different energies to differentiate between soft tissue and bone. The X-rays are directed anterior–posterior or vice versa, depending on the instrument. Fan-beam and pencil-beam machines can scan laterally around the side of a patient, and are useful to measure the bone density of the lumbar spine.

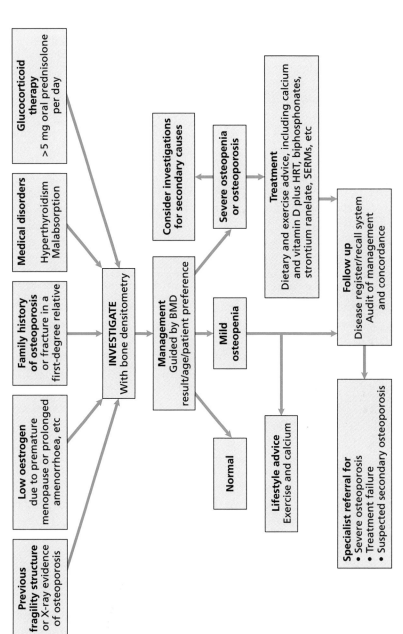

Figure 5.1 Flow chart for the management of osteoporosis

Values for bone mineral density (BMD) may be quoted as g/cm^2 or converted into values that relate to the average young normal female (or male) peak bone mass or to the bone mass related to the patient's age group. These are T scores and Z scores, respectively, and are calculated as follows:

- T score $= \dfrac{\text{Patient's BMD} - \text{population peak BMD}}{\text{Standard deviation (SD) of population peak BMD}}$

- Z score $= \dfrac{\text{Patient's BMD} - \text{population age-related BMD}}{\text{SD of population age-related BMD}}$

In women, peak density of the lumbar spine is reached around the middle of the third decade of life. According to the WHO (1994), osteoporosis is diagnosed if the T score is –2.5 or lower (see above). Values can be plotted on a chart to show the mean and limits of +2 or –2 SD of a healthy population (Figure 5.2).

Calibrations for average bone densities are often based on a US database of the upper femur, called the National Health and Nutrition Examination Survey (NHANES) database.

The main sites for measurement are the spine (L1 or L2–L4) and various regions of interest at the hip. Some difficulties are encountered in measuring the spine. This occurs especially in the elderly where osteophytes due to osteoarthritis, kyphosis, scoliosis and aortic calcification can lead to falsely increased values of BMD. It is now recommended, therefore, that the best site to measure for diagnosis is the hip. Bone mineral density of the 'total hip' and the neck of femur are the most commonly used measurements.

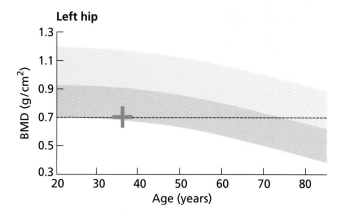

Figure 5.2 Femoral neck bone density showing mean and limits of +2 and –2 standard deviations of a healthy population

Peripheral DXA (pDXA) systems are also available to measure the forearm or calcaneus and may be considered to be a risk assessment tool. They cannot replace hip DXA, however, for the formal diagnosis of osteoporosis.

Generally agreed indications for densitometry are as follows:

- any oestrogen-deficient postmenopausal woman who would want to be treated or would want to continue treatment if found to be osteopenic or osteoporotic
- patients older than 50 years suspected to be osteoporotic on radiography or clinically through height loss or low-impact fracture, such as Colles' radial fracture or fracture of any peripheral bone excluding the digits
- patients who have a medical condition that predisposes to osteoporosis if effective treatment is available – for example, metabolic bone disease, thyroid disease, liver disease, anorexia nervosa, malabsorption syndromes and other rarer causes of osteoporosis
- patients who use systemic corticosteroids with a dose of >5 mg pred-nisolone or equivalent for a projected duration of 3 months or longer
- oestrogen-deficient women younger than 45 years who experience primary amenorrhoea or secondary amenorrhoea (including that resulting from hysterectomy)
- patients with a family history of fracture, particularly hip fracture, in a first-degree relative.

The frequency of follow-up scans for those at risk of osteoporosis or those being treated for established disease is controversial. Initially, follow-up scans may be undertaken at 2 years to assess response to treatment and, in general, should not be done more frequently than every 3 years thereafter. Most private healthcare plans in the USA provide coverage for BMD testing to monitor the therapeutic response to therapy, but they will not generally reimburse testing for this indication more often than every 2 years. When BMD is measured by densitometry, atom for atom, strontium attenuates X-rays more strongly than calcium, as it has a higher atomic number (calcium 20, strontium 38), a fact that can lead to an overestimation of the BMD value. The use of bone markers may replace DXA for early assessment of response to treatment.

Quantitative ultrasound

This technique involves the transmission of a low-amplitude ultrasound beam, usually through the calcaneus, and measures bone strength. It has the attraction of being portable and not using ionizing radiation. It remains to be evaluated fully before it can be used in routine clinical practice. In terms of diagnostic capability, most data involve prediction of fractures in elderly women, in whom it seems to be a competent measure of the risk of hip fracture. It remains to be determined, however, whether it can predict fracture at other sites or in younger menopausal women.

Single-energy X-ray absorptiometry

This method is used commonly for wrist scans.

Quantitative computed tomography

This method provides measurement of the spine, hip and wrist. It does not have a diagnostic ability superior to that of DXA. Its use in clinical practice is limited by poorer precision and much higher radiation doses than used with DXA.

Biochemical markers of bone metabolism

Over the last decade, our ability to detect the subtle changes in bone turnover associated with postmenopausal bone loss and osteoporosis has been enhanced by the development of specific and sensitive markers of this process. Biochemical markers of bone turnover are classified as markers of resorption or formation. It should be remembered, however, that bone resorption and formation are 'coupled' processes, and therefore, in most situations, any marker can be used to determine the overall rate of bone turnover.

Most markers of bone resorption are products of collagen degradation that are released into the circulation and finally excreted in the urine. Tartrate-resistant acid phosphatase is secreted by osteoclasts, and its levels are measured in serum.

Markers of bone formation are by-products of collagen formation, matrix proteins or enzymes associated with osteoblast activity (Table 5.1). A potential use of these markers is to monitor anti-osteoporotic therapy, as they will show changes within 3–6 months, while DXA will take more than one year. These markers, however, are not universally available for routine use.

Predicting fracture

The FRAX tool has been developed by the WHO to evaluate fracture risk. It is based on individual patient models that integrate the risks associated with clinical risk factors as well as femoral neck BMD. The clinical risk factors comprise BMI as a continuous variable, a prior history of fracture, a parental history of hip fracture, use of oral glucocorticoids, rheumatoid arthritis and

Table 5.1

Most commonly used biochemical markers of bone turnover

Bone formation	Bone resorption
By-products of collagen synthesis • Pro-collagen type 1 C terminal pro-peptide (PICP)* • Pro-collagen type 1 N terminal pro-peptide (PINP)* Matrix protein • Osteocalcin (OC) Osteoblast enzyme • Total alkaline phosphatase (total ALP)* • Bone alkaline phosphatase (bone ALP)*	Collagen degradation products • Hydroxyproline (Hyp)[†] • Pyridinoline (PYD)*[†] • Deoxypyridinoline (DPD)*[†] Cross-linked telopeptides of type I collagen • N-terminal cross-linked telopeptide (NTX)*[†] • C-terminal cross-linked telopeptide (CTX)*[†] • C-terminal cross-linked telopeptide generated by matrix metalloproteinases (MMPs) (CTX-MMP, formerly ICTP)* Osteoclast enzyme • Tartrate-resistant acid phosphatase (TRACP)*

* Measured in serum. [†] Measured in urine
Adapted from Hannon (2003)

other secondary causes of osteoporosis, current smoking, and alcohol intake of 3 or more units daily.

The FRAX models have been developed from studying population-based cohorts from Europe, North America, Asia and Australia.

The FRAX algorithms give the 10-year probability of hip and other major osteoporotic fractures.

Risk factors for cardiovascular disease

Lipid and lipoprotein measurements

A number of guidelines have been published, as elevated cholesterol levels are associated with increased risk of coronary heart disease (CHD), and lipid-lowering agents such as statins have been shown to be effective in primary and secondary prevention trials. However, there are differences between the genders. In women, the benefits of statins are mainly found in secondary, rather than primary, prevention trials; cholesterol levels change over time differently in men and women (men reach their peak cholesterol level at about age 50, and women at about age 60); low-density lipoprotein cholesterol (LDL-C) is less predictive and high-density lipoprotein cholesterol (HDL-C) is more predictive of CHD risk in women.

There are various recommendations for screening for hyperlipidaemia in women. In the USA, the National Cholesterol Education Program (NCEP) recommends screening all women older than 20 years with a fasting lipid profile (total cholesterol, LDL and HDL) at least every 5 years. However, the US Preventive Services recommend screening those who are at higher risk and in whom treatment decisions might change as a result of the screening. Thus, while they recommend routine screening for lipid disorders in women aged over 45, screening in younger women is recommended only if they have other risk factors for CHD. In the UK, the Joint British Societies' guidelines (JBS 2) on cardiovascular disease (CVD) prevention in clinical practice recommend that prevention should focus equally on (i) people with established atherosclerotic CVD, (ii) people with diabetes, and (iii) apparently healthy individuals at high risk (CVD risk of ≥20% over 10 years) of developing symptomatic atherosclerotic disease with gender-specific predictions. All adults from 40 years onwards who have no history of CVD or diabetes and who are not already on treatment for blood pressure or lipids should be considered for an opportunistic comprehensive CVD risk assessment in primary care. Younger adults (<40 years) with a family history of premature atherosclerotic disease should also have their cardiovascular risk factors measured.

Optimal levels for women are LDL-C of <2.6 mmol/l (<100 mg/dl), triglycerides of <1.7 mmol/l (<150 mg/dl), HDL-C of >1.3 mmol/l (>50 mg/dl), and non-HDL-C of <3.38 mmol/l (<130 mg/dl). For women with established CVD or diabetes, LDL-C levels should be <2.0 mmol/l (<77 mg/dl).

With regard to prandial status, a 12-hour fast is essential for triglyceride measurement and calculated LDL, but not for total or HDL-C measurements.

Homocysteine

Despite the evidence linking elevated plasma homocysteine levels to CVD, the value of population screening is debated. Testing should be limited to screening patients considered high risk, such as those with a personal or family history of premature atherosclerosis and those with renal failure.

Mammography and genetic testing

Mammography screening programmes

Screening programmes vary throughout the world. In the UK, the National Health Service Breast Screening Programme (NHSBSP) offers mammograms every 3 years to women aged 50–70 years. Screening is also available for older women, but there is no automatic invitation.

Screening in high-risk women

Familial breast cancer

In the UK, the National Institute for Health and Clinical Excellence (NICE) has produced clinical guidance for the classification and care of women at risk of familial breast cancer in primary, secondary and tertiary care:

- Women at or near population risk of developing breast cancer (that is, a 10-year risk of less than 3% for women aged 40–49 years and a lifetime risk of less than 17%) are cared for in primary care.
- Women at raised risk of developing breast cancer (that is, a 10-year risk of 3–8% for women aged 40–49 years or a lifetime risk of 17% or greater but less than 30%) are generally cared for in secondary care.
- Women at high risk of developing breast cancer (that is, a 10-year risk of greater than 8% for women aged 40–49 years or a lifetime risk of 30% or greater) are cared for in tertiary care. High risk also includes an individual risk of 20% or greater chance of a faulty *BRCA1*, *BRCA2* or *TP53* gene in the family with these mutations.

For the purpose of these calculations, a woman's age should be assumed to be 40 years for a woman in her 40s. A 10-year risk should then be calculated for the age range 40–49 years.

Women who meet the criteria in Box 5.1 should be offered referral to secondary or tertiary care, as appropriate. NICE has also produced guidelines for mammographic and magnetic resonance imaging (MRI) surveillance (Table 5.2) in high-risk women.

Long-term survivors of Hodgkin's disease

Long-term follow-up of Hodgkin's disease (HD) survivors has revealed an increased incidence of secondary malignancy. The relative risk of breast cancer after supradiaphragmatic irradiation (SDI) or mantle radiotherapy is significantly increased, predominantly in those under the age of 30 years at the time of irradiation. Studies have shown a relative risk of 15–25, with greater risks for those treated between the ages of 10 and 16 years. The median induction

Box 5.1

Clinical guidance for the classification and care of women at risk of fmailial breast cancer in primary, secondary and tertiary care (Adapted from NICE, 2006)

Criteria for referral to secondary and tertiary care
Refer to secondary care if:
- one first-degree female relative diagnosed with breast cancer at younger than age 40 years, or
- one first-degree male relative diagnosed with breast cancer at any age, or
- one first-degree relative with bilateral breast cancer where the first primary was diagnosed at younger than age 50 years

or
- two first-degree relatives, or one first-degree and one second-degree relative, diagnosed with breast cancer at any age, or
- one first-degree or second-degree relative diagnosed with breast cancer at any age and one first-degree or second-degree relative diagnosed with ovarian cancer at any age (one of these should be a first-degree relative)

or
- three first-degree or second-degree relatives diagnosed with breast cancer at any age

Advice should be sought from the designated secondary care contact if any of the following are present in the family history, in addition to breast cancers in relatives not fulfilling the above criteria:

➢ bilateral breast cancer
➢ male breast cancer
➢ ovarian cancer
➢ Jewish ancestry
➢ sarcoma in a relative younger than age 45 years
➢ glioma or childhood adrenal cortical carcinoma
➢ complicated patterns of multiple cancers at a young age
➢ paternal history of breast cancer (two or more relatives on the father's side of the family)

Refer to tertiary care if:
- At least the following female breast cancers only in the family:
  ○ two first-degree or second-degree relatives diagnosed with breast cancer at younger than an average age of 50 years (at least one must be a first-degree relative), or
  ○ three first-degree or second-degree relatives diagnosed with breast cancer at younger than an average age of 60 years (at least one must be a first-degree relative), or
  ○ four relatives diagnosed with breast cancer at any age (at least one must be a first-degree relative)

or
- Families containing one relative with ovarian cancer at any age and, on the same side of the family:
  ○ one first-degree relative (including the relative with ovarian cancer) or second-degree relative diagnosed with breast cancer at younger than age 50 years, or

- two first-degree or second-degree relatives diagnosed with breast cancer at younger than an average age of 60 years, or
- another ovarian cancer at any age

or

- Families containing bilateral cancer (each breast cancer has the same count value as one relative):
  - one first-degree relative with cancer diagnosed in both breasts at younger than an average age of 50 years, or
  - one first-degree or second-degree relative diagnosed with bilateral breast cancer and one first-degree or second-degree relative diagnosed with breast cancer at younger than an average age of 60 years

or

- Families containing male breast cancer at any age and on the same side of the family, at least:
  - one first-degree or second-degree relative diagnosed with breast cancer at younger than age 50 years, or
  - two first-degree or second-degree relatives diagnosed with breast cancer at younger than an average age of 60 years

or

- A formal risk assessment has given risk estimates of:
  - a 20% or greater chance of a *BRCA1*, *BRCA2* or *TP53* mutation being harboured in the family, or
  - a greater than 8% chance of developing breast cancer at age 40–49 years, or
  - a 30% or greater lifetime risk of developing breast cancer

Clinicians should seek further advice from a specialist genetics service for families containing any of the following, in addition to breast cancers:

- ➢ Jewish ancestry
- ➢ sarcoma in a relative younger than age 45 years
- ➢ glioma or childhood adrenal cortical carcinomas
- ➢ complicated patterns of multiple cancers at a young age
- ➢ very strong paternal history (four relatives diagnosed at younger than 60 years of age on the father's side of the family)

All affected relatives must be on the same side of the family and must be blood relatives of the woman and each other

In cases of bilateral breast cancer, each breast cancer has the same count value as one relative

Key

First-degree relatives:	mother, father, daughter, son, sister, brother
Second-degree relatives:	grandparent, grandchild, aunt, uncle, niece and nephew; half-sister and half-brother
Third-degree relatives:	great-grandparent, great-grandchild, great-aunt, great-uncle, first cousin, grand-nephew and grand-niece

Table 5.2

Guidelines for mammographic and MRI surveillance (Adapted from NICE, 2006)

Age (years)	Mammography	MRI
20–29	Should not be available for women younger than age 30 years	Should be available only for those at exceptionally high risk (that is, annual risk of ≥1%; for example, *TP53* carriers
30–39	Should be available to women satisfying referral criteria for secondary or specialist care only as part of a research study (ethically approved) or nationally approved and audited service Individualized strategies should be developed for exceptional cases, such as women from families with *BRCA1*, *BRCA2* and *TP53* mutations (or women with equally high risk)	Should be available annually to: • women with a 10-year risk of greater than 8% • *BRCA1*, *BRCA2* or *TP53* mutation carriers • women who have not been tested but have a high chance of carrying a *BRCA1* or *TP53* mutation, specifically: – those at 50% risk of carrying a *BRCA1* or *TP53* mutation in a tested family – those at 50% risk of carrying *BRCA1* or *TP53* mutation from untested or inconclusively tested families with at least 60% risk of *BRCA1* or *TP53* mutation (that is, 30% chance of carrying a mutation themselves)
40–49	Should be available annually to women at raised and high risk satisfying referral criteria for secondary or specialist care	Should be available annually to: • women with 10-year risk of greater than 20% • women with 10-year risk of greater than 12% whose mammography has shown a dense breast pattern[a] • *TP53*, *BRCA1* and *BRCA2* mutation carriers • Women who have not been tested but have high chance of carrying a *BRCA1* or *TP53* mutation, specifically: – those at 50% risk of carrying *BRCA1* or *TP53* mutation in a tested family – those at 50% risk of carrying *BRCA1* or *TP53* mutation from untested or inconclusively tested families with at least 60% risk of *BRCA1* or *TP53* mutation (that is, 30% chance of carrying a mutation themselves)

50+	Should be available every 3 years as part of the NHS Breast Screening Programme	Should not be available for women older than 50 years
	More frequent mammographic surveillance should take place only as part of a research study (ethically approved) or nationally approved and audited service	
	Individualized strategies should be developed for exceptional cases, such as women from families with *BRCA1*, *BRCA2* or *TP53* mutations (or women at equally high risk)	

[a] As defined by the three-point mammographic classification used by UK breast radiologists (Breast Group of the Royal College of Radiologists, 1989). Supporting information: An 8% risk aged 30–39 years and a 12% risk aged 40–49 years would be run by women with the following family histories:

2 close relatives diagnosed with average age <30 years[b]

3 close relatives diagnosed with average age <40 years[b]

4 close relatives diagnosed with average age <50 years[b]

[b] All relatives must be on the same side of the family and one must be a mother or sister of the consultee.

A genetic test would usually be required to determine a 10-year risk of 20% or greater in women aged 40–49 years.

For the purposes of these calculations, a woman's age should be assumed to be 30 years for a woman in her 30s and 40 years for a woman in her 40s. A 10-year risk should then be calculated for the periods 30–39 years and 40–49 years, respectively.

period for breast cancer following SDI for HD in adults is long, around 15 years (range 4–20). However, this may be shorter in patients treated in childhood. Surveillance programmes have been proposed (Table 5.3).

Factors affecting mammographic density

There is strong evidence that mammographic breast density is an independent risk factor for breast cancer, denser tissue on imaging being a marker of susceptibility. It is positively associated with stromal (ie non-epithelial breast cells) and epithelial cells and negatively associated with fat. It is hypothesized that mammographic breast density reflects genetic and environmental factors influencing the proliferation and quantity of stromal and epithelial tissue. This could explain the fact that in age-matched women, individual breast density can vary widely. Increased breast density can reduce the sensitivity and specificity of mammography.

Table 5.3

Surveillance for women at risk of breast cancer after treatment for Hodgkin's disease with supradiaphragmatic irradiation (Adapted from Ralleigh, 2005)

Age (years)	Recommended surveillance	
<25	*No imaging*	
25–29	*Annual MRI* but if contraindications *annual ultrasound* (mammography is not recommended for this age group)	
30–50	*Baseline two-view mammogram.* Women should then be divided into two groups:	
	Predominantly fatty breast tissue	**Dense breast tissue**
	Annual two-view mammography	*Annual two-view mammography plus MRI:* Unless there are contraindications when the patient should be offered *Annual mammography plus ultrasound*: If breast tissue becomes predominantly fatty prior to the age of 50 years the patient should move into group 1 (i.e. annual mammography only)
>50	*Three-yearly mammography* should be offered within the NHS Breast Screening Programme (NHSBSP)	

Effect of exogenous hormones

Exogenous hormones can affect mammographic density, and the effects differ with individual preparations. The response of breast tissue to exogenous hormones may be predictive of future development of breast cancer.

HRT

Placebo-controlled, randomized trials (ie the Women's Health Initiative [WHI] and Progestin Oestrogen–Progestin Intervention [PEPI] studies) have shown that unopposed oestrogen (ie conjugated equine oestrogen 0.625 mg) does not increase mammographic density, but combined therapy (both cyclical and continuous combined, irrespective of the class of progestogen) does in about one in four women who take it within the first year of exposure. The individual degree of density increase is in the order of 3–6%. There is no evidence that duration of use influences this effect. Evidence from the WHI study suggests that a change in mammographic density with combined HRT was not predictive of an abnormal mammogram (ie one that would generate recommendation for further evaluation). This study also showed that while density was unaffected with unopposed conjugated equine oestrogens, the risk of women diagnosed with a mammographic abnormality was increased, although this mainly resulted in a recommendation for short-term follow-up only (ie benign change).

There are few data on the effect of oestradiol on mammographic breast density.

The Million Women Study and observational evidence report that HRT (both unopposed and combined) increases the risk of interval breast cancers – that is, cancers diagnosed between mammographic screens due to reduced sensitivity (ie being missed at a previous screen). Evidence suggests that HRT is associated with a higher risk of a missed diagnosis due to a reduction in mammographic sensitivity and would be expected if combined HRT increases density in some women. Risk of interval cancers would be expected to be less with unopposed oestrogen, as this does not have a significant effect on density. In the WHI study there was a reduction in diagnosed cancers in women allocated to receive conjugated equine oestrogens that persisted for the duration of follow-up (ie 7 years). This would argue against an increase in interval cancer rate due to missed cancers or inappropriate reassurance from short-term follow-up.

Withdrawal of HRT before mammography has been reported to result in regression of increases in density associated with HRT sufficient to enable more accurate film reading. In the combined HRT component of the WHI study, where women who used HRT were advised to stop their therapy for 3 months before randomization, no difference was seen in the proportion of abnormal mammograms at baseline, an observation that supports a screening benefit for withdrawal of HRT. This question has not been subject to controlled evaluation, but observational data suggest that this regression of density can occur in as little as 2 weeks. Evidence is insufficient at present to recommend this for women using HRT who require a mammogram for surveillance or diagnostic purposes.

Overall, given that about 50% of HRT users in the UK use unopposed therapy, the WHI and PEPI trials suggest the majority of women currently using HRT in the UK who attend the NHSBSP are unlikely to develop any increase in breast density that could in turn influence mammographic sensitivity.

Tibolone

Tibolone does not increase mammographic breast density and while it reduces the risk of breast cancer in women aged over 60 by 68%, it is associated with a significant increase in recurrence in breast cancer survivors. This is a good illustration that changes or lack of change in mammographic density with hormonal exposure cannot be directly correlated with future breast cancer risk.

Tamoxifen and raloxifene

Both tamoxifen and raloxifene are associated with a decrease in mammographic breast density of the order of about 10%. The reduction in breast cancer diagnosis with both these hormonal agents is about 40–50%.

Genetic testing

Familial cancer services have been developed in many countries in response to a rapidly evolving demand for genetic counselling and testing for breast cancer risk. The lifetime risk (to 85 years of age) of developing breast cancer in developed countries worldwide is 11% (one in nine). Twenty-seven per cent of women are estimated to have an inherited predisposition to breast cancer, but only 3–5% are likely to carry gene faults that entail a substantially increased risk (ie >50%). Most breast cancers arise in women without a family history and are termed sporadic. In women with a family history (6–19%), this familial association can be the result of chance, environmental factors or genetic predisposition. An inherited risk is likely if the woman has a family member with a young age of onset, or has a family with a cluster of cases and a history of bilateral disease. Inherited mutations that affect the BRCA1 and BRCA2 genes have been identified and have an associated lifetime risk of breast cancer of 80%. They account for about one-third of inherited breast cancers. Patients with breast cancer from families who carry mutations have a high risk of cancer in the other breast (>50% by the age of 70 years). The lifetime risk of subsequent ovarian cancer also is increased: up to 60% for women with BRCA1 and up to 40% for women with BRCA2. A very small proportion (<1%) of breast cancers are associated with rarer cancer predisposition syndromes and germline mutations in genes such as *TP53* in Li-Fraumeni syndrome or *PTEN* in Cowden syndrome. Other, as yet unidentified, inherited gene mutations are likely. Breast cancer genes can be inherited through both sexes; family members may transmit these genes without developing cancer themselves (that is, penetrance is variable).

An appropriate screening programme for women with *BRCA1* or *BRCA2* mutations and consequently high risk of ovarian cancer includes transvaginal ultrasound scan, with or without colour Doppler imaging, in combination with serum CA125 measurements. However, there is no definitive evidence that surveillance can reduce mortality.

In the absence of any effective chemoprevention strategies, prophylactic mastectomy is the only option available for preventing breast cancer in known mutation carriers. Although this reduces mortality from breast cancer significantly, it does not completely reduce the risk of breast cancer, as some breast tissue may be left behind. Trials are under way to assess the role of tamoxifen and aromatase inhibitors in the chemoprevention of breast cancer in women at high risk. Breast cancers associated with *BRCA1* often do not express hormone receptors, so endocrine chemoprevention may be ineffective.

Endometrial assessment

Postmenopausal bleeding and abnormal perimenopausal bleeding are important clinical problems in both users and non-users of HRT. The main onus is to exclude carcinoma of the endometrium or cervix and premalignant endometrial hyperplasia (Figures 5.3 and 5.4).

When should the endometrium be assessed?

HRT non-users
Abnormal bleeding, such as postmenopausal bleeding, a sudden change in menstrual pattern, intermenstrual bleeding or postcoital bleeding, requires investigation. Many countries have rapid access services for women with postmenopausal bleeding.

HRT users
With sequential HRT, abnormal bleeding is denoted by a change in pattern of withdrawal bleeding or breakthrough bleeding. In women taking continuous combined or long-cycle regimens, breakthrough bleeding that persists for more than 4–6 months or does not lessen requires assessment. Similarly, women who bleed after amenorrhoea while taking a continuous combined

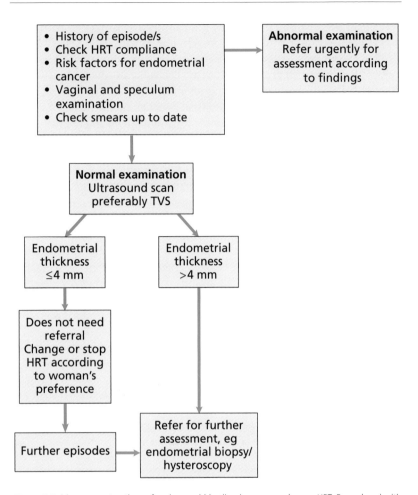

Figure 5.3 Management pathway for abnormal bleeding in women who use HRT. Reproduced with permission from Oehler (2003)

regimen need evaluation. There is no need, however, to assess the endometrium routinely before starting HRT in women with no abnormal bleeding, as the incidence of endometrial cancer is less than one per 1000 (<0.1%).

Relevant risk factors for endometrial cancer should be sought in the history. These include obesity, diabetes, nulliparity, history of chronic anovulation (eg polycystic ovary syndrome), late menopause, use of unopposed oestrogens or tamoxifen, and family history of hereditary nonpolyposis colorectal, ovarian, or endometrial cancers.

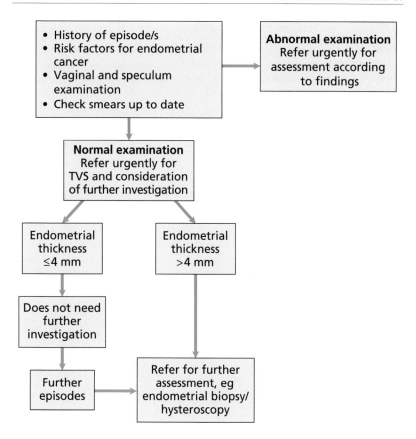

Figure 5.4 Management pathway for abnormal bleeding in women who do not use HRT. Reproduced with permission from Oehler (2003)

Methods of assessment

Clinical assessment

Speculum and bimanual examination with visualization of the cervix should be undertaken. Cervical cytology should be up to date in accordance with local screening programmes. In HRT users, the type of treatment should be documented, as should concordance with treatment – for example, missed tablets or non-adherent patches that ultimately may be implicated in the abnormal bleeding.

Transvaginal ultrasound scanning

Transvaginal ultrasound scanning (TVS) is used for initial assessment. TVS-initiated triage has substantial cost savings versus biopsy-based algorithms in evaluating typical populations of postmenopausal women with abnormal vaginal bleeding. It measures endometrial thickness and also gives information on other pelvic disorder, such as fibroids and ovarian cysts. However, it does not give a histological diagnosis. A thickened endometrium or a cavity filled with fluid indicates an increased risk of malignancy or other disorder (hyperplasia or polyps). Detection of benign lesions, such as endometrial polyps and submucous fibroids, can be enhanced by sonohysterography with instillation of saline into the uterine cavity. Use of this technique varies worldwide.

Endometrial thickness cut-off values

Premenopausally, total anteroposterior thickness (both endometrial layers) varies from 4 to 8 mm in the proliferative phase and peaks at 8–16 mm during the secretory phase. Some debate remains on whether or not a cut-off value of 3, 4 or 5 mm should be used in postmenopausal women who do and do not use HRT: 4 mm may be preferred, as 10-year follow-up data are available. It must be remembered that endometrial thickness in women who take sequential HRT varies depending on the phase of therapy (oestrogen alone or oestrogen combined with progestogen). It is thus preferable to perform TVS after the bleeding has ceased and before the combined oestrogen plus progestogen phase is started. In women who take continuous combined regimens, women who use the Mirena coil to provide the progestogen, and women who do not use HRT, however, TVS can be performed at any time.

Endometrial biopsy

The principal purpose of endometrial biopsy is to obtain a histological diagnosis. Two main techniques are used: aspiration curettage as an outpatient procedure and dilation and curettage (D&C) under anaesthetic. No existing method will sample the entire uterine cavity. In most cases, therefore, endometrial biopsy has to be complementary to other techniques, such as TVS or hysteroscopy, to increase sensitivity.

The advantage of aspiration curettage is that it avoids general anaesthesia and has fewer complications than D&C, such as bleeding and uterine perforation. Various instruments with narrow cannulas for endometrial biopsy are available: a commonly used device is the Pipelle. This device obtains an adequate endometrial specimen in up to 99% of women, and a meta-analysis found that it has a detection rate of 99.6% for endometrial carcinoma in postmenopausal women.

Endometrial histology

Proliferative and secretory changes are reported in endometrium removed from premenopausal women. In the case of endometrial hyperplasia, the situation is more complicated, because several classifications have been used over the years. The only important distinction in prognostic and therapeutic terms is between hyperplasias that are associated with a significant risk of progressing into an endometrial adenocarcinoma and those devoid of such risk. The WHO classification has four categories:

1. simple hyperplasia
2. complex hyperplasia
3. simple atypical hyperplasia
4. complex atypical hyperplasia.

Progression from hyperplasia to cancer has been reported to occur in only 1–3% of patients with hyperplasia without atypia. Hyperplasia with cytological atypia, however, has significant potential for malignant change, which has been shown to occur in 28% of patients over an average of 13.4 years. Furthermore, it can coexist with endometrial cancer.

Hysteroscopy
Hysteroscopy allows direct visualization of the uterine cavity. It is a superior method for the detection of endometrial polyps and submucosal myomas, which can easily be missed by endometrial biopsy procedures, ultrasonography or 'blind' curettage. Diagnostic hysteroscopy can be performed as an outpatient procedure without anaesthetic or as a formal theatre procedure.

Hysteroscopy has been advocated by many as the standard for the diagnosis of abnormal uterine bleeding, but it is not 100% accurate, and lesions can be missed. A systematic quantitative review found that the diagnostic accuracy of hysteroscopy is high for endometrial cancer but only moderate for non-malignant or premalignant endometrial disease.

In addition, caution is advised in the uncritical use of hysteroscopy in patients suspected of having endometrial cancer. Single-case reports have shown the hysteroscopic dissemination of viable malignant cells into the abdominal cavity from uteri containing an endometrial carcinoma. How frequently this occurs and whether or not it has any prognostic impact remains unknown.

Persistent bleeding

A dilemma exists if there is a negative initial endometrial sampling and the abnormal bleeding persists. Due to the risk of a sampling error, repeated TVS and biopsy are recommended in patients with persistent symptoms.

Further reading

Endocrine investigations

Davis SR, Davison SK, Donath S, *et al.* Circulating androgen levels and self-reported sexual function in women. *JAMA* 2005;**294**:91–6.

Hall JE. Neuroendocrine changes with reproductive aging in women. *Semin Reprod Med* 2007;**25**:344–51.

Parker S. Follicle stimulating hormone: facts and fallacies. *J Br Menopause Soc* 2004;**10**:166–8.

Slater CC, Hodis HN, Mack WJ, *et al.* Markedly elevated levels of estrone sulfate after long-term oral, but not transdermal, administration of estradiol in postmenopausal women. *Menopause* 2001;**8**:200–3.

Skeletal assessment

Blake GM, Lewiecki EM, Kendler DL, Fogelman I. A review of strontium ranelate and its effect on DXA scans. *J Clin Densitom* 2007;**10**:113–19.

Bonnick SL, Shulman L. Monitoring osteoporosis therapy: bone mineral density, bone turnover markers, or both? *Am J Med* 2006;**119**(Suppl 1):S25–31.

FRAX – WHO Fracture Risk Assessment Tool. www.shef.ac.uk/FRAX.

Hannon RA, Eastell R. Biochemical markers of bone turnover and fracture prediction. *J Br Menopause Soc* 2003;**9**:10–15.

Johnell O. The socioeconomic burden of fractures: today and in the 21st century. *Am J Med* 1997;**103**:S20–5.

Johnell O, Kanis J. Epidemiology of osteoporotic fractures. *Osteoporos Int* 2005;**16**(Suppl 2):S3–7.

Kanis JA, Johnell O, Oden A, *et al.* FRAX and the assessment of fracture probability in men and women from the UK. *Osteoporos Int* 2008;**19**:385–97.

NIH Consensus Development Panel on Osteoporosis Prevention, Diagnosis, and Therapy. Osteoporosis prevention, diagnosis, and therapy. *JAMA* 2001;**285**:785–95.

Poole KES, Compston JE. Osteoporosis and its management. *BMJ* 2006;**333**:1251–6.

Ralston SH. Genetics of osteoporosis. *Proc Nutr Soc* 2007;**66**:158–65.

Scholes D, LaCroix AZ, Ichikawa LE, *et al.* Change in bone mineral density among adolescent women using and discontinuing depot medroxyprogesterone acetate contraception. *Arch Pediatr Adolesc Med* 2005;**159**:139–44.

Walsh JS, Eastell R, Peel NF. Effects of depot medroxyprogesterone acetate on bone density and bone metabolism before and after peak bone mass: a case-control study. *J Clin Endocrinol Metab* 2008;**93**:1317–23.

World Health Organization. Assessment of fracture risk and its application to screening for postmenopausal osteoporosis. WHO Technical Report Series 843. Geneva: WHO, 1994.

Risk factors for cardiovascular disease

Chamberlain KL. Homocysteine and cardiovascular disease: a review of current recommendations for screening and treatment. *J Am Acad Nurse Pract* 2005;**17**:90–5.

Expert Executive Summary of the Third Report of the National Cholesterol Education Program (NCEP) Expert Panel on Detection, Evaluation, and Treatment of High Blood Cholesterol in Adults (Adult Treatment Panel III). *JAMA* 2001;**285**:2486–97.

JBS 2: Joint British Societies' Guidelines on Prevention of Cardiovascular Disease in Clinical Practice. *Heart* 2005;**91**(Suppl 5):v1–52.

Mosca L, Appel LJ, Benjamin EJ, *et al.* Summary of the American Heart Association's evidence-based guidelines for cardiovascular disease prevention in women. *Arterioscler Thromb Vasc Biol* 2004;**24**:394–6.

Mosca L, Banka CL, Benjamin EJ, *et al.* Evidence-based guidelines for cardiovascular disease prevention in women: 2007 update. *J Am Coll Cardiol* 2007;**49**:1230–50.

Prospective Studies Collaboration; Lewington S, Whitlock G, Clarke R, *et al.* Blood cholesterol and vascular mortality by age, sex, and blood pressure: a meta-analysis of individual data from 61 prospective studies with 55,000 vascular deaths. *Lancet* 2007;**370**:1829–39.

Walsh JM. Lipids in women: screening and treatment. *J Am Med Womens Assoc* 2003;**58**:240–7.

Walsh JM, Pignone M. Drug treatment of hyperlipidemia in women. *JAMA* 2004;**291**: 2243–52.

Mammography and genetic screening

Banks E, Reeves G, Beral V, *et al.* Impact of use of hormone replacement therapy on false positive recall in the NHS breast screening programme: results from the Million Women Study. *BMJ* 2004;**328**:1291–2.

Blanks RG, Wallis MG, Moss SM. A comparison of cancer detection rates achieved by breast cancer screening programmes by number of readers, for one and two view mammography: results from the UK National Health Service breast screening programme. *J Med Screen* 1998;**5**:195–201.

Boyd NF, Guo H, Martin LJ, *et al.* Mammographic density and the risk and detection of breast cancer. *N Engl J Med* 2007;**356**:227–36.

Bruce D, Robinson J, McWilliams S, *et al.* Long-term effects of tibolone on mammographic density. *Fertil Steril* 2004;**82**:1343–7.

Chlebowski RT, Anderson G, Pettinger M, *et al.* Estrogen plus progestin and breast cancer detection by means of mammography and breast biopsy. *Arch Intern Med* 2008;**168**:370–7.

Chlebowski RT, Hendrix SL, Langer RD, *et al.* Influence of estrogen plus progestin on breast cancer and mammography in healthy postmenopausal women. The Women's Health Initiative randomized trial. *JAMA* 2003;**289**:3243–53.

Colacurci N, Fornaro F, De Franciscis P, *et al.* Effects of a short-term suspension of hormone replacement therapy on mammographic density. *Fertil Steril* 2001;**76**: 451–5.

Cuzick J, Powles T, Veronesi U, *et al.* Overview of the main outcomes in breast-cancer prevention trials. *Lancet* 2003;**361**:296–300.

Daling JR, Malone KE, Doody DR, *et al.* Association of regimens of hormone replacement therapy to prognostic factors among women diagnosed with breast cancer aged 50–64 years. *Cancer Epidemiol Biomarkers Prev* 2003;**12**:1175–81.

Eilertsen AL, Karssemeijer N, Skaane P, *et al.* Differential impact of conventional and low-dose oral hormone therapy, tibolone and raloxifene on mammographic breast density, assessed by an automated quantitative method. *BJOG* 2008;**115**:773–9.

Greendale GA, Reboussin BA, Sie A, *et al.* Effects of estrogen and estrogen-progestin on mammographic parenchymal density. Postmenopausal Estrogen/Progestin Interventions (PEPI) Investigators. *Ann Intern Med* 1999;**130**:262–9.

Greendale GA, Reboussin BA, Slone S, *et al.* Postmenopausal hormone therapy and change in mammographic density. *J Natl Cancer Inst* 2003;**95**:30–7.

Gronwald J, Tung N, Foulkes WD, *et al.*; Hereditary Breast Cancer Clinical Study Group. Tamoxifen and contralateral breast cancer in *BRCA1* and *BRCA2* carriers: an update. *Int J Cancer* 2006;**118**:2281–4.

Harvey JA, Pinkerton JV, Herman CR. Short-term cessation of hormone replacement therapy and improvement of mammographic specificity. *J Natl Cancer Inst* 1997;**89**:1623–5.

Hofling M, Lundström E, Azavedo E, *et al.* Testosterone addition during menopausal hormone therapy: effects on mammographic breast density. *Climacteric* 2007;**10**:155–63.

Lichtenstein P, Holm N, Verkasalo P, *et al.* Environmental and heritable factors in the causation of cancer – analyses of cohorts of twins from Sweden, Denmark, and Finland. *N Engl J Med* 2000;**343**:78–85.

Lynch HT, Silva E, Snyder C, Lynch JF. Hereditary breast cancer. I. Diagnosing hereditary breast cancer syndromes. *Breast J* 2008;**14**:3–13.

Meiser B, Gaff C, Julian-Reynier C, *et al.* International perspectives on genetic counseling and testing for breast cancer risk. *Breast Dis* 2006–7;**27**:109–25.

National Institute for Clinical Excellence. Familial Breast Cancer. Clinical Guideline 41. October 2006. www.nice.org.uk/guidance/cg41.

McTiernan A, Martin CF, Peck JD, *et al.*; Women's Health Initiative Mammogram Density Study Investigators. Estrogen-plus-progestin use and mammographic density in postmenopausal women: Women's Health Initiative Randomized Trial. *J Natl Cancer Inst* 2005;**97**:1366–76.

Nelson HD, Huffman LH, Fu R, Harris EL; US Preventive Services Task Force. Genetic risk assessment and *BRCA* mutation testing for breast and ovarian cancer susceptibility: systematic evidence review for the US Preventive Services Task Force. *Ann Intern Med* 2005;**143**:362–79.

Pavelka JC, Li AJ, Karlan BY. Hereditary ovarian cancer – assessing risk and prevention strategies. *Obstet Gynecol Clin North Am* 2007;**34**:651–65, vii–viii.

Ralleigh G. Screening for breast cancer in women with previous mantle radiotherapy for Hodgkin's disease. *Breast Cancer Online* 2005;**8**:1–5, e52.

Stefanick ML, Anderson GL, Margolis KL, *et al.* Effects of conjugated equine estrogens on breast cancer and mammography screening in postmenopausal women with hysterectomy. *JAMA* 2006;**295**:1647–57.

Rutter CM, Mandelson MT, Laya MB, *et al*. Changes in breast density associated with initiation, discontinuation, and continuing use of hormone replacement therapy. *JAMA* 2001;**285**:171–6.

Stallard S, Litherland JC, Cordiner CM, *et al*. Effect of hormone replacement therapy on the pathological stage of breast cancer: population based cross-sectional study. *BMJ* 2000;**320**:348–9.

Sterns EE, Zee B. Mammographic density changes in perimenopausal and post-menopausal women: is effect of hormone replacement therapy predictable? *Breast Cancer Res Treat* 2000;**59**:125–32.

Endometrial assessment

Affinito P, Palomba S, Sammartino A, *et al*. Ultrasonographic endometrial monitoring during continuous-sequential hormonal replacement therapy regimen in postmenopausal women. *Maturitas* 2001;**39**:239–44.

Arikan G, Reich O, Weiss U, *et al*. Are endometrial carcinoma cells disseminated at hysteroscopy functionally viable? *Gynecol Oncol* 2001;**83**:221–6.

Clark TJ, Voit D, Gupta JK, *et al*. Accuracy of hysteroscopy in the diagnosis of endometrial cancer and hyperplasia: a systematic quantitative review. *JAMA* 2002;**288**:1610–21.

Clark TJ, Neelakantan D, Gupta JK. The management of endometrial hyperplasia: an evaluation of current practice. *Eur J Obstet Gynecol Reprod Biol* 2006;**125**:259–64.

Dijkhuizen FP, Mol BW, Brolmann HA, Heintz AP. The accuracy of endometrial sampling in the diagnosis of patients with endometrial carcinoma and hyperplasia: a meta-analysis. *Cancer* 2000;**89**:1765–72.

Epstein E, Ramirez A, Skoog L, Valentin L. Dilatation and curettage fails to detect most focal lesions in the uterine cavity in women with postmenopausal bleeding. *Acta Obstet Gynecol Scand* 2001;**80**:1131–6.

Epstein E, Ramirez A, Skoog L, Valentin L. Transvaginal sonography, saline contrast sonohysterography and hysteroscopy for the investigation of women with post-menopausal bleeding and endometrium >5 mm. *Ultrasound Obstet Gynecol* 2001;**18**:157–62.

Gull B, Karlsson B, Milsom I, Granberg S. Can ultrasound replace dilation and curettage? A longitudinal evaluation of postmenopausal bleeding and transvaginal sonographic measurement of the endometrium as predictors of endometrial cancer. *Am J Obstet Gynecol* 2003;**188**:401–8.

Gupta JK, Chien PF, Voit D, *et al*. Ultrasonographic endometrial thickness for diagnosing endometrial pathology in women with postmenopausal bleeding: a meta-analysis. *Acta Obstet Gynecol Scand* 2002;**81**:799–816.

Kurman RJ, Kaminski PF, Norris HJ. The behavior of endometrial hyperplasia. A long-term study of 'untreated' hyperplasia in 170 patients. *Cancer* 1985;**56**: 403–12.

Lacey JV Jr, Ioffe OB, Ronnett BM, *et al*. Endometrial carcinoma risk among women diagnosed with endometrial hyperplasia: the 34-year experience in a large health plan. *Br J Cancer* 2008;**98**:45–53.

Medverd JR, Dubinsky TJ. Cost analysis model: US versus endometrial biopsy in evaluation of peri- and postmenopausal abnormal vaginal bleeding. *Radiology* 2002;**222**:619–27.

Rutqvist LE, Johansson H; Stockholm Breast Cancer Study Group. Long-term follow-up of the randomized Stockholm trial on adjuvant tamoxifen among postmenopausal patients with early stage breast cancer. *Acta Oncol* 2007;**46**:133–45.

Sankaranarayanan R, Gaffikin L, Jacob M, *et al.* A critical assessment of screening methods for cervical neoplasia. *Int J Gynaecol Obstet* 2005;**89**(Suppl 2): S4–12.

Scottish Intercollegiate Guidelines Network. Investigation of post-menopausal bleeding. Guideline no. 61. www.sign.ac.uk.

Smith-Bindman R, Kerlikowske K, Feldstein VA, *et al.* Endovaginal ultrasound to exclude endometrial cancer and other endometrial abnormalities. *JAMA* 1998;**280**:1510–17.

Timmermans A, van Doorn LC, Opmeer BC, *et al.*; Dutch Study in Postmenopausal Bleeding (DUPOMEB). Follow-up of women after a first episode of postmenopausal bleeding and endometrial thickness greater than 4 millimeters. *Obstet Gynecol* 2008;**111**:137–43.

Van Doorn HC, Timmermans A, Opmeer BC, *et al.* What is the recurrence rate of postmenopausal bleeding in women who have a thin endometrium during a first episode of postmenopausal bleeding? *Acta Obstet Gynecol Scand* 2008;**87**:89–93.

Weiderpass E, Persson I, Adami HO, *et al.* Body size in different periods of life, diabetes mellitus, hypertension, and risk of postmenopausal endometrial cancer (Sweden). *Cancer Causes Control* 2000;**11**:185–92.

MANAGEMENT STRATEGIES

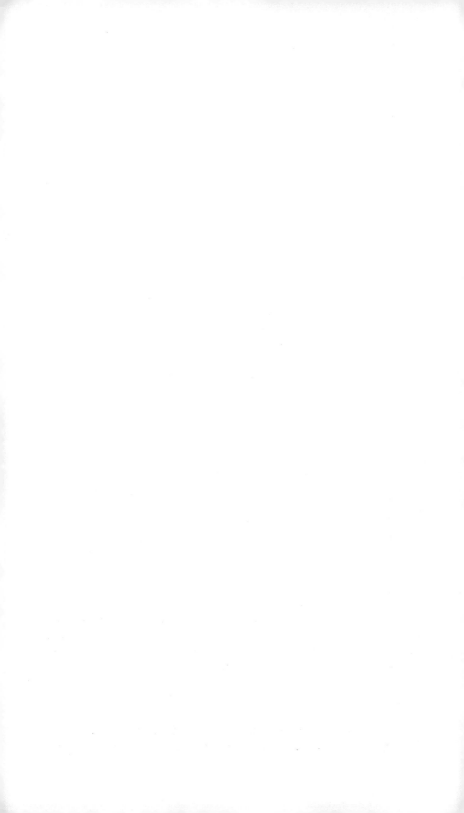

6 Oestrogen-based therapies

At present, more than 50 oestrogen-based preparations, which feature different strengths, combinations and routes of administration, are licensed worldwide. Various terms are used: hormone replacement therapy (HRT), hormone therapy (HT), oestrogen therapy (ET) and oestrogen and progestogen therapy (EPT) for combined preparations – whether sequential or continuous combined.

Components of hormone replacement therapy

Hormone replacement therapy consists of an oestrogen combined with a progestogen in non-hysterectomized women. Progestogens are given cyclically or continuously with the oestrogen. Different routes of administration are employed: oral, transdermal, subcutaneous and vaginal.

Oestrogens

Two types of oestrogen are available: synthetic and natural. Synthetic oestrogens, such as ethinyl oestradiol, are generally considered to be unsuitable for

HRT because of their greater metabolic impact, apart from use in young women with premature ovarian failure. Natural oestrogens include oestradiol, oestrone and oestriol, which, although chemically synthesized from soybeans or yams, are molecularly identical to the natural human hormone. Conjugated equine oestrogens contain about 50–65% oestrone sulphate, and the remainder consists of equine oestrogens – mainly equilin sulphate. These also may be classified as 'natural'. Much confusion surrounds what constitutes a 'natural' oestrogen. In this book, we have taken the view that a 'natural' oestrogen is one that is found in normal physiology irrespective of whether it has been prepared by chemical synthesis or extraction from a plant or animal source.

The generally accepted minimum bone-sparing doses of oestrogen are listed below (Table 6.1), although increasing evidence shows that even lower doses may be effective. Although these also may improve vasomotor symptoms, oestrogenic side-effects may be reduced. Young women who experience a surgical menopause, however, initially may need higher doses of oestrogen to alleviate menopausal symptoms. Conversely, older women usually require lower doses to control their symptoms.

Progestogens

The progestogens used in HRT are almost all synthetic, are structurally different from progesterone, and are also derived from plant sources. Currently, they are used mainly in tablet form, although norethisterone and levonorgestrel are available in transdermal patches combined with oestradiol, and levonorgestrel can be delivered directly to the uterus (Box 6.1). The native molecule progesterone is formulated as an oral tablet or a 4% vaginal gel and is licensed for use in HRT, but its availability varies worldwide. A progesterone pessary to be used vaginally or rectally is available, but this is currently not licensed for HRT.

Table 6.1

Minimum bone-sparing doses of HRT

HRT	Dose
Oestradiol oral	1–2 mg
Oestradiol patch	25–50 μg
Oestradiol gel	1–5 g*
Oestradiol implant	50 mg every 6 months
Conjugated equine oestrogens	0.3–0.625 μg daily

*Depends on preparation

Box 6.1

Classification of progestogens

Progestogens structurally related to progesterone
1 Pregnane derivatives:
    (a) acetylated (also called 17α-hydroxyprogesterone derivatives): medroxy-progesterone acetate, megestrol acetate, cyproterone acetate)
    (b) non-acetylated: dydrogesterone
2 19-Norpregnane derivatives (also called 19-norprogesterone derivatives):
    (a) acetylated: nomegestrol acetate
    (b) non-acetylated: trimegestone

Progestogens structurally related to testosterone (also called 19-nortestosterone derivatives)
1 Ethinylated:
    (a) oestranes: norethisterone, ethynodiol diacetate
    (b) gonanes: levonorgestrel, norgestrel, desogestrel, gestodene, norgestimate
2 Non-ethinylated: dienogest, drospirenone

Tibolone

Tibolone is a synthetic steroid compound that is itself inert, but, on absorption, it is converted *in vivo* to metabolites with oestrogenic, progestogenic and androgenic actions. It is used in postmenopausal women who wish to have amenorrhoea. Classified as HRT in the *British National Formulary*, it is used to treat vasomotor, psychological and libido problems. The daily dose is 2.5 mg. It conserves bone mass, and reduces the risk of vertebral and non-vertebral, but not hip, fractures.

Androgens

Testosterone implants and patches may be used to improve libido but are not successful in all women, as other factors, such as marital problems, may be involved. Testosterone patches have the advantage of an easily reversible delivery system, as implants cannot be easily removed.

Delivery systems

Oral versus parenteral administration

The main consideration in route of administration is whether to use oral or non-oral delivery. The latter avoids the gut and first-pass effects on the liver. After oral administration, the predominant circulating oestrogen is oestrone; after parenteral administration, it is oestradiol.

Substances normally synthesized in the liver may be affected differentially by oral or parenteral delivery. For example, high doses of conjugated equine oestrogens increase the production of renin substrate, but the type of substrate induced is not the one normally associated with hypertension. The clinical significance is unclear, as blood pressure does not normally increase with this form of HRT. Oral oestrogen also induces the hepatic production and release of sex hormone binding globulin. Furthermore, production of certain coagulation factors and lipids may be affected differentially by the route of administration.

Extensive debate currently surrounds the relative merits of the oral route versus the non-oral route. At present, the transdermal route seems to have no clear advantage over the oral route for the majority of women. However transdermal oestrogen confers a lower risk of venous thromboembolism and gallbladder disease (see Chapter 7). Furthermore, all oestrogens, regardless of the route of administration, eventually pass through the liver and are recycled by the enterohepatic circulation. In routine clinical practice, therefore, the oral route is the usual first line of treatment unless the patient has a pre-existing medical condition. Some practitioners, however, prefer to embark on transdermal treatment on the grounds that it mimics the natural route of oestrogen delivery in premenopausal women – when oestrogen is delivered from the ovaries directly into the venous system.

Non-oral delivery systems

Transdermal systems: patch and gel

Oestradiol and progestogens can diffuse through the skin. Two transdermal systems are available: patch and gel. Two patch technologies exist: alcohol-based reservoir patches, which have an adhesive outer ring, and matrix patches, in which the hormone is distributed evenly throughout the adhesive. Skin reactions are less common with matrix patches than with reservoir patches. Of the progestogens, currently only norethisterone and levonorgestrel are delivered transdermally in patches. At present, only oestradiol is delivered in a gel.

Implants

Oestradiol implants are crystalline pellets of oestradiol that are inserted subcutaneously under local anaesthetic and release oestradiol over many months. Implants have the advantage that once inserted patients do not have to remember to take their drugs. A significant concern is tachyphylaxis, which may be defined as a recurrence of menopausal symptoms while the implant is still releasing adequate levels of oestradiol. Another concern is that implants may remain effective for many years and cannot easily be removed.

A check on levels of oestradiol before reimplantation should be considered, especially in women who return more frequently for treatment, to ensure that the preimplantation level is in the normal premenopausal range (<1000 pmol/l).

Intrauterine systems

Originally used to provide contraception, the intrauterine system delivers 20 μg/day of levonorgestrel to the endometrium and can provide the progestogen component of HRT. The oestrogen then can be given orally or transdermally. This system also provides a solution to the problem of contraception in the perimenopause and is also the only way in which a 'no bleed' regimen can be achieved in perimenopausal women. A device that releases 10 μg/day is being evaluated for early postmenopausal women.

Hysterectomized women

In general, hysterectomized women should be given oestrogen alone and have no need for a progestogen. Furthermore, combined HRT may entail a greater risk of breast cancer than oestrogen alone (see Chapter 7). Concern about a remnant of endometrium in the cervical stump may exist in women who have had a subtotal hysterectomy. If this is suspected to be the case, the presence or absence of bleeding induced by monthly sequential HRT may be a useful diagnostic test.

Non-hysterectomized women

Progestogens are added to oestrogens to reduce the increased risk of endometrial hyperplasia and carcinoma, which occurs with unopposed oestrogen; they need not be given to women who have undergone hysterectomy. Progestogen can be given 'sequentially' for 10–14 days every 4 weeks, for 14 days every 13 weeks, or every day – that is, 'continuously'. The first leads to monthly bleeds, the second to bleeds every 3 months, and the last aims to achieve amenorrhoea. Progestogen must be given to women who have undergone endometrial ablative techniques, as it cannot be assumed that all the endometrium has been removed – even if prolonged amenorrhoea has been achieved.

Perimenopausal women

The options available are monthly cyclic or 3-monthly cyclic regimens. For women with infrequent menstruation and those who are intolerant of progestogens, a 3-monthly preparation can be considered. Only one is available in the UK at present: it contains oestradiol valerate and medroxyproges-terone acetate. Continuous combined regimens should not be used in peri-menopausal women because of the high risk of irregular bleeding.

Postmenopausal women

By strict definition, women are considered to be postmenopausal 12 months after their last menstrual period. In clinical practice, however, the definition is difficult to apply, especially in women who started HRT in the peri-menopause. Although monthly and 3-monthly cyclic or continuous combined regimens can be used in postmenopausal women, the last are more popular because of the lack of induced bleeding. Furthermore, continuous combined treatment may have a reduced risk of endometrial cancer compared with sequential regimens (see Chapter 7). Continuous combined therapy induces endometrial atrophy.

Irregular bleeding or spotting can occur during the first 4–6 months of continuous combined therapy and does not warrant investigation. Endometrial assessment needs to be considered if the bleeding becomes heavier rather than lighter, if it persists beyond 6 months, or if it occurs after a significant time of amenorrhoea (see Chapter 5). The incidence of irregular bleeding may be reduced by increasing the ratio of the progestogen to the oestrogen.

Switching from sequential to continuous combined therapy

It may be difficult to decide when women can switch from sequential to continuous combined therapy. Pragmatically, postmenopausal status can be estimated from the following factors:

- *Age*: it has been estimated that 80% of women will be postmenopausal by the age of 54 years.
- *Previous amenorrhoea or increased levels of follicle-stimulating hormone (FSH)*: women who experienced 6 months of amenorrhoea or had increased levels of FSH in their mid-40s are likely to be postmenopausal after taking several years of monthly sequential HRT.

Starting systemic hormone replacement therapy

Symptoms of oestrogen deficiency, such as hot flushes, mood changes, tiredness, arthralgia and vaginal dryness, may start several months or years before periods stop: such a history in women older than 40 years is a classic presentation. Amenorrhoea need not be awaited before HRT is started. The dose used should control the individual's menopausal symptoms, and control of symptoms can be used to establish the minimum required dose.

Managing the side-effects of systemic hormone replacement therapy

Side-effects can be related to oestrogen or progestogen, or a combination of both. Many of the so-called side-effects of HRT, in fact, are start-up effects consequent on administration of oestrogen, which previously had been lacking. Furthermore, side-effects are more likely to be problematic in women who have been deficient in oestrogen for a long period. It is essential, therefore, to discuss early effects, such as breast tenderness, at the outset and to explain that they usually resolve by 3 months into treatment. If unprepared for start-up effects, women will be alarmed and may well stop HRT. Usually, it is possible to determine whether the side-effects are oestrogenic (occurring continuously or randomly throughout the cycle) or progestogenic (occurring in a cyclical pattern during the progestogen phase of sequential HRT).

Side-effects

Oestrogen-related side-effects include fluid retention, bloating, breast tenderness or enlargement, nausea, headaches, leg cramps and dyspepsia.

Progestogen-related side-effects are fluid retention, breast tenderness, headaches or migraine, mood swings, depression, acne, lower abdominal pain and backache.

Complaints of weight gain and poor cycle control are common to both elements.

Management strategies

Management strategies that are useful in clinical practice will be described; interestingly, none have been examined systematically in clinical trials.

Oestrogen-related side-effects

Transient side-effects

Side-effects are often transient and resolve without any change in treatment with increasing duration of use. Patients should be encouraged to persist with therapy for about 12 weeks to await resolution. The analogy with certain symptoms of early pregnancy may be useful. Patients can be reassured and given appropriate advice in order to minimize these problems.

Breast tenderness may be alleviated by addition of gamolenic acid. Leg cramps can improve with lifestyle changes. Nausea or gastric upset with oral preparations may be alleviated by adjusting the timing of the dose or taking the dose with food; lactose sensitivity should be considered.

Persistent side-effects
With persistent side-effects, the options include the following:

• *Reduce dose* – when doing this, the endpoints of treatment, such as symptom control and the prevention of osteoporosis, must be borne in mind.
• *Change oestrogen type* – oestradiol or conjugated equine oestrogens.
• *Change route of delivery* – oral, patch, gel or implant.

Progestogen-related side-effects

Progestogenic side-effects are more problematic because of the need to provide endometrial protection. They are connected to type, duration and dose of progestogen. Once again, perseverance with therapy should be encouraged, as hysterectomy must be considered only as a last resort. Useful strategies include the following:

• *Change the type of progestogen* – for example, from a 19-nortestosterone to a 17-hydroxyprogesterone derivative.
• *Reduce the dose* – but not below the recommended levels for endometrial protection.
• *Change the administration route*, using transdermal, vaginal or intrauterine progesterone or progestogen.
• *Reduce the duration*, as progestogens can be taken for 10–14 days of each monthly sequential regimen.
• *Reduce the frequency*, using long-cycle HRT that administers progestogen for 14 days every 3 months (but this is suitable only for women without natural regular cycles).

Continuous combined therapy often reduces progestogenic side-effects with established use, but it is suitable only for postmenopausal women.

Weight gain

Weight gain is often given as a major reason why women are reluctant to start or continue treatment. Randomized, placebo-controlled trials, however, repeatedly show no evidence of HRT-induced weight gain.

Bleeding

Monthly sequential regimens should produce regular predictable and acceptable bleeding, starting towards the end or soon after the end of the progestogen phase. Non-concordance with therapy, drug interactions (such as antiepileptics and herbal remedies) or gastrointestinal upset, which can interfere with absorption, need to be excluded. Pelvic pathology will need exclusion if the problem persists or does not respond to treatment (see Chapter 5). Useful strategies include the following:

- Increase dose or change type of progestogen in women with heavy or prolonged bleeding.
- Increase dose or change type of progestogen in women with bleeding early in the progestogen phase.
- Change type of progestogen in women with painful bleeding.
- Change regimen or increase progestogen in women with irregular bleeding.

No bleeding reflects an atrophic endometrium and occurs in 5% of women, but pregnancy needs to be excluded in perimenopausal women or those with early ovarian failure. Breakthrough bleeding is common in the first 3–6 months of continuous combined and long-cycle HRT regimens, but if it continues thereafter, it should be investigated as for postmenopausal bleeding (see Chapter 5).

Duration of systemic therapy

The duration of systemic therapy depends on the endpoints of treatment.

Treatment of vasomotor symptoms

Treatment for vasomotor symptoms should be continued for up to 5 years and then stopped to evaluate whether or not they have recurred. This duration will not significantly increase the risk of breast cancer (see Chapter 7). Although menopausal symptoms usually resolve within 2–5 years, some women experience symptoms for many years – even into their 70s and 80s (see Chapter 2)

Prevention or treatment of osteoporosis

For this issue, treatment needs to be continued for life, as bone mineral density falls when treatment is stopped. Use of HRT for 5–10 years after the menopause has been assumed to delay the peak incidence of hip fracture by a corresponding amount. If the median age of hip fracture is 79 years, therefore, and if this is delayed by 5–10 years through the use of HRT, most women would not live long enough to suffer a hip fracture. Most epidemiological evidence, however, suggests that 5–10 years of HRT soon after the menopause does not give any significant reduction in the risk of hip fracture 30 years later (see Chapter 7). Although some women will be happy to take HRT for life, others may view treatment as a continuum of options and will wish to change to other agents, such as a bisphosphonate or strontium ranelate, because of the small but measurable increase in risk of breast cancer associated with the long-term use of combined HRT.

Premature menopause

In this case, women are usually advised to continue with HRT until the average age of the natural menopause – that is, 52 years (see Chapter 12). Thereafter, the issues discussed in the above sections are relevant.

Stopping systemic hormone replacement therapy

Various strategies are used, but they have not been examined in clinical trials. The limited evidence available shows no clear advantage of stopping gradually or abruptly. The main issue is a recurrence of menopausal symptoms, such as flushes and myalgia, on stopping, as has been reported by participants of the Women's Health Initiative, who discontinued HRT suddenly. Anecdotally, older women need less oestrogen to control their symptoms, and thus a lower dose can be tried before stopping. Although alternate-day, or even less frequent, oral treatment can be used in hysterectomized women, concerns exist that this strategy could lead to irregular bleeding or insufficient addition of progestogen in women whose uterus is intact.

Treatment of local symptoms

Some women do not wish to take, or cannot tolerate, systemic HRT and simply require relief of local symptoms, which usually are urogenital. Local treatment options include low-dose natural oestrogens, such as vaginal oestradiol by tablet or ring or oestriol by cream or pessary. Creams and pessaries may affect condom integrity. Conjugated equine oestrogen (CEE) cream is also available, but this is well absorbed from the vagina and can cause endometrial stimulation. Systemic absorption with oestradiol vaginal tablets or ring is low without systemic effects, and hormone levels remain within the postmenopausal range. Thus, if the recommended topical oestradiol and oestriol preparations are used, there is no need to add a progestogen for endometrial protection. However, if CEEs are used on a long-term basis, a progestogen should be taken for endometrial protection. Vaginal oestrogens can also be used with systemic oestrogens. Oestriol can also be given orally, but only in hysterectomized women because of the increased risk of endometrial cancer.

Bio-identical hormones

In some countries, an alternative approach to menopause management and postmenopausal health is the use of 'natural' or 'bio-identical' hormones. In the USA, the Food and Drug Administration (FDA) is concerned about the claims for safety, effectiveness, and superiority of preparations that are made in compounding pharmacies.

Further reading

Bachmann G, Lobo RA, Gut R, *et al.* Efficacy of low-dose oestradiol vaginal tablets in the treatment of atrophic vaginitis: a randomized controlled trial. *Obstet Gynecol* 2008;**111**:67–76.

CKS. Clinical topic – Menopause. cks.library.nhs.uk/menopause.

Cummings SR. LIFT study is discontinued. *BMJ* 2006;**332**:667.

Ettinger B, Ensrud KE, Wallace R, *et al.* Effects of ultralow-dose transdermal estradiol on bone mineral density: a randomized clinical trial. *Obstet Gynecol* 2004;**104**: 443–51.

Grady D, Sawaya GF. Discontinuation of postmenopausal hormone therapy. *Am J Med* 2005;**118**(Suppl 12B):163–5.

Hampton N, Rees MC, Barlow DH, *et al.* Levonorgestrel intrauterine system (LNG-IUS) with conjugated oral equine estrogen: a successful regimen for HRT in perimenopausal women. *Hum Reprod* 2005;**20**:2653–60.

Haskell SG. After the Women's Health Initiative: postmenopausal women's experiences with discontinuing estrogen replacement therapy. *J Womens Health* 2004;**13**: 438–42.

Heikkinen J, Vaheri R, Timonen U. A 10-year follow-up of postmenopausal women on long-term continuous combined hormone replacement therapy: update of safety and quality-of-life findings. *J Br Menopause Soc* 2006;**12**:115–25.

Hope S. Myalgia after stopping hormone replacement therapy. *J Br Menopause Soc* 2004;**10**:126.

Kingsberg S. Testosterone treatment for hypoactive sexual desire disorder in postmenopausal women. *J Sex Med* 2007;**4**(Suppl 3):227–34.

Kuehn BM. FDA warns claims for pharmacy-made 'bio-identical' hormones are misleading. *JAMA* 2008;**299**:512.

Nelson HD. Commonly used types of postmenopausal estrogen for treatment of hot flashes: scientific review. *JAMA* 2004;**291**:1610–20.

Notelovitz M, Funk S, Nanavati N, Mazzeo M. Estradiol absorption from vaginal tablets in postmenopausal women. *Obstet Gynecol* 2002;**99**:556–62.

Ockene JK, Barad DH, Cochrane BB, *et al.* Symptom experience after discontinuing use of estrogen plus progestin. *JAMA* 2005;**294**:183–93.

Prestwood KM, Kenny AM, Kleppinger A, Kulldorff M. Ultralow-dose micronized 17beta-estradiol and bone density and bone metabolism in older women: a randomized controlled trial. *JAMA* 2003;**290**:1042–8.

Rioux JE, Devlin C, Gelfand MM, *et al*. 17beta-estradiol vaginal tablet versus conjugated equine estrogen vaginal cream to relieve menopausal atrophic vaginitis. *Menopause* 2000;**7**:156–61.

Simunic V, Banovic I, Ciglar S, *et al*. Local estrogen treatment in patients with urogenital symptoms. *Int J Gynaecol Obstet* 2003;**82**:187–97.

Slater CC, Hodis HN, Mack WJ, *et al*. Markedly elevated levels of estrone sulfate after long-term oral, but not transdermal, administration of estradiol in postmenopausal women. *Menopause* 2001;**8**:200–3.

Sturdee DW, Rantala ML, Colau JC, *et al*. The acceptability of a small intrauterine progestogen-releasing system for continuous combined hormone therapy in early postmenopausal women. *Climacteric* 2004;**7**:404–11.

Suckling J, Lethaby A, Kennedy R. Local oestrogen for vaginal atrophy in postmenopausal women. *Cochrane Database Syst Rev* 2003;**4**:CD001500.

Thakar R, Ayers S, Clarkson P, *et al*. Outcomes after total versus subtotal abdominal hysterectomy. *N Engl J Med* 2002;**347**:1318–25.

Waaseth M, Bakken K, Dumeaux V, *et al*. Hormone replacement therapy use and plasma levels of sex hormones in the Norwegian Women and Cancer Postgenome Cohort – a cross-sectional analysis. *BMC Womens Health* 2008;**8**:1.

Weisberg E, Ayton R, Darling G, *et al*. Endometrial and vaginal effects of low-dose estradiol delivered by vaginal ring or vaginal tablet. *Climacteric* 2005;**8**:83–92.

7 Benefits, risks and uncertainties of oestrogen-based therapy

> Women's Health Initiative and Million Women Study
> Benefits of hormone replacement therapy
> Risks of hormone replacement therapy
> Uncertainties
> Further reading

Publication of the results of the Women's Health Initiative (WHI) and Million Women Study (MWS) since 2002 has led to considerable uncertainties among health professionals and women about the role of hormone replacement therapy (HRT). This chapter will discuss the benefits, risks and uncertainties of oestrogen-based HRT, as well as of tibolone, as it has oestrogenic properties.

Women's Health Initiative and Million Women Study

Women's Health Initiative

The WHI is a large, complex series of clinical investigations, designed in the early 1990s, of strategies for the primary prevention and control of some of the most common causes of morbidity and mortality among healthy, postmenopausal women aged 50–79. It consisted of a randomized, controlled trial and an observational study. The randomized trial considered not only HRT but also calcium and vitamin D supplementation and diets with low-fat content (Box 7.1). If eligible, women could choose to enrol in one, two, or all three of the randomized trial components. The randomized trial involved 68,132 women (mean age 63 years) trying conjugated equine oestrogens (0.625 mg) alone ($n = 10{,}739$), conjugated equine oestrogens (0.625 mg) in combination with medroxyprogesterone acetate (2.5 mg) ($n = 16{,}608$), a low-fat eating pattern ($n = 48{,}835$) and calcium and vitamin D supplementation ($n = 36{,}282$). Clinical trial screenees ($n = 93{,}676$) who were ineligible or unwilling to participate in the controlled trial were recruited into an observational study that assessed new risk indicators and biomarkers for disease. The WHI Extension Study is following up 115,400 participants from each of the original WHI study components until 2010.

Box 7.1

Interventions evaluated by Women's Health Initiative clinical trial

---

Hormone replacement therapy (unopposed and combined) – hypothesized to reduce the risk of coronary heart disease (CHD) and other cardiovascular diseases and, secondarily, to reduce the risk of hip and other fractures, with increased risk of breast cancer being studied as a possible adverse outcome

Low-fat eating pattern – hypothesized to prevent breast cancer and colorectal cancer and, secondarily, to prevent CHD

Supplementation with calcium and vitamin D – hypothesized to prevent hip fractures and, secondarily, to prevent other fractures and colorectal cancer

---

Million Women Study

The observational MWS has provided information about a diverse range of HRT regimens with the exception of vaginal preparations from women aged 50–64 (mean age 57) attending the NHS Breast Screening Programme (NHSBSP) in the UK. A total of 1,084,110 women were recruited between 1996 and 2001; about half had ever used HRT. The average duration of follow-up was 2.6 years.

However, several publications have questioned the design, analysis and conclusions of both these studies. The results of the MWS should be interpreted in the context of placebo-controlled HRT trials and the knowledge that the data provided are probably representative of about 25% of all women in the UK in the 50–64-year age group (based on uptake for the first, prevalent NHSBSP round of 75%, MWS questionnaire completion in attendees of 50%, and the number of UK screening centres that participated in the study [66 out of 94]). Differences between women attending or not attending the NHSBSP and between attendees who agreed or declined to participate in the study cannot be easily controlled for.

Benefits of hormone replacement therapy

Benefits

Vasomotor symptoms
There is good evidence from randomized, placebo-controlled studies, including the WHI, that oestrogen is effective in treating hot flushes, and improvement is usually noted within 4 weeks. It is more effective than non-hormonal preparations such as clonidine and selective serotonin reuptake inhibitors (see Chapter 8). Maximum therapeutic response to any particular formulation is

usually achieved by 3 months. Relief of vasomotor symptoms is the most common indication for HRT prescription and is often used for less than 5 years. Oestrogen dose needs to be tailored to the severity of symptoms; lower doses than used previously may be sufficient.

Urogenital symptoms and sexuality

Symptoms such as vaginal dryness, soreness, superficial dyspareunia, and urinary frequency and urgency respond well to oestrogens, which may be given either topically or systemically. Improvement may take several months. Recurrent urinary tract infections may be prevented by vaginal but not oral oestrogen replacement. Topical oestrogens may have a weak effect on urinary urge incontinence, but no improvement of stress incontinence.

Long-term treatment is often required, as symptoms can recur on cessation of therapy. Sexuality may be improved with oestrogen alone but may also need testosterone addition, especially in young, oophorectomized women (see Chapter 6).

Osteoporosis

There is evidence from randomized, controlled trials (including the WHI) that HRT reduces the risk of both spine and hip as well as other osteoporotic fractures. The 'standard' bone-conserving doses of oestrogen were previously considered to be oestradiol 2 mg, conjugated equine oestrogens 0.625 mg, and transdermal 50 μg oestradiol patch. However, it is now evident that lower doses may also conserve bone mass. Epidemiological studies suggest that, for HRT to be an effective method of preventing fracture, continuous and lifelong use is required. However, it has now been shown that just a few years' treatment with HRT around the time of menopause may have a long-term effect on fracture reduction. Regulatory authorities have advised that HRT should not be used as a first-line treatment to prevent osteoporosis, as the risks outweigh the benefits. This conclusion has been vigorously challenged. While alternatives to HRT use are available for the prevention and treatment of osteoporosis in elderly women, oestrogen still remains the best option, particularly in younger (under 60) and/or symptomatic women. Few data are available on the efficacy of alternatives such as bisphosphonates in women with premature ovarian failure. Currently, HRT is significantly cheaper to prescribe than alternative therapies such as bisphosphonates, strontium ranelate and parathyroid hormone. Unlike HRT, there are no data suggesting that bisphosphonates reduce fracture risk in women with normal bone density.

Colorectal cancer

Results from the oestrogen progestogen arm, but not the oestrogen alone arm, of the WHI study concur with observational studies that HRT reduces the risk of colorectal cancer. However, little is known about the colorectal cancer risk when treatment is stopped. There is no information about HRT in high-risk populations, and current data do not allow prevention as a recommendation.

Risks of hormone replacement therapy

Breast cancer

Hormone replacement therapy appears to entail a similar degree of risk to that associated with late natural menopause (2.3% compared with 2.8% per year respectively). In their 1997 reanalysis of worldwide observational data, the Collaborative Group on Hormonal Factors in Breast Cancer suggested that current use of any HRT for more than 5 years will increase breast cancer risk if started in the 50+ age group (ie relative risk [RR] 1.35, 95% confidence interval [CI] 1.20–1.49). In absolute numbers, this equates to two extra breast cancers per 1000 women who use HRT from the age of 50 for 5 years. Such an effect is not seen in women who start HRT early for premature menopause, indicating that it is the duration of lifetime sex hormone exposure that is relevant.

Addition of progestogen increases breast cancer risk compared with oestrogen alone, but this has to be balanced against the reduction in risk of endometrial cancer provided by combined therapy (see section on endometrial cancer). Intuitively, lower doses of steroids should be associated with reduced risk of breast cancer, but there are no epidemiological data to support this. Irrespective of the type of HRT prescribed, breast cancer risk falls after cessation of use, risk being no greater than that in women who have never been exposed to HRT after 5 years. The increased risk of breast cancer with longer-term exposure, however, seems to be limited in most studies to lean women (ie BMI <25 kg/m^2). Moreover, the increased risk of breast cancer with HRT is low and similar to the risk entailed by obesity, alcohol intake over 2 units per day, and nulliparity or late age at first full-term pregnancy, and is lower than that entailed by certain inherited genetic mutations or mantle radiotherapy (Table 7.1).

The WHI found that:

- The risk of breast cancer in the oestrogen-alone arm of the WHI study was lower than in the placebo group. Risk of breast cancer was significantly reduced in women with no previous exposure at entry.
- In the combined arm, there was evidence of a duration effect with an increase in risk beginning to emerge 3 years after randomization but only in women with a history of HRT use prior to study entry.

Breast cancer risk. Adapted from American Cancer Society (2007–08)

Relative risk (RR)	Risk factor
High risk (RR >4)	Certain inherited genetic mutations, eg *BRCA1* or *BRCA2*
	Personal history breast cancer
	Biopsy confirmed atypical hyperplasia*
	High-dose radiation to chest (mantle radiotherapy for Hodgkin's disease at age <35 years)
Moderate risk (RR 2–4)	Family history (see Chapter 5)
Low increased risk (RR 1.1–2)	Benign breast disease without evidence of epithelial atypia
	Recent and long-term use of HRT
	Late age at first full-term pregnancy (>30 years)
	Early menarche (<12 years)
	Late menopause (>55 years)
	Nulliparity
	Alcohol consumption
	Postmenopausal obesity
	High socio-economic status
	Height (tall)
	Jewish heritage

*This is a risk marker; ie risk of subsequent breast cancer affects both breasts (Chapter 12)

The MWS found that:

- Risk increased with all HRT regimens (ie unopposed oestrogen and combined HRT), in contrast to the WHI and a large observational study that found no increased risk with unopposed oestrogen.
- The greatest degree of risk was with combined HRT, and it was not influenced by route of administration.
- Different oestrogens or progestogens did not appear to alter risk, nor did the pattern of progestogen administration (ie cyclical or continuous).

The higher risk estimates reported in the MWS than in the randomized WHI study, especially the oestrogen-alone arm, which found a reduced risk, probably reflect the observational nature of the MWS and suggest that the latter study has probably overestimated the risk of breast cancer. The reported increase in breast cancer risk in the MWS after an apparently short duration of exposure (ie less than 1–2 years) can be attributed to an underestimation of the total duration of HRT exposure, as the risk estimates presented were based on HRT use at recruitment. The study investigators did not adjust the total duration of use to account for the likely continued use of HRT in the period between recruitment and cancer diagnosis (ie mean of 1.2 years). An immediate risk is unlikely, since it is generally thought that the effect of HRT on breast cancer is primarily on growth promotion rather than initiation of a new tumour. Furthermore, the finding of a complete disappearance of breast cancer risk within 14 months of HRT withdrawal, even after long-term therapy, is biologically implausible.

Breast cancer mortality

Breast cancer mortality is the most important outcome. It is unlikely that any randomized trials, including WHI, will ever be large enough to evaluate this endpoint reliably. Advice about the effect of HRT on breast cancer survival has to be drawn from observational studies and/or predictions of outcome based on the biological characteristics of tumours. Overall, observational studies suggest that HRT has no significant effect on survival compared with non-users. The MWS reported an increased mortality in current HRT users, but this was of borderline significance, and in the absence of information about tumour pathology, stage and treatment, it is difficult to draw any definitive conclusions. The increased mortality may simply reflect the fact that a greater number of cancers were detected in HRT users.

In the WHI study, combined HRT-associated tumours were, on average, 2 mm larger than placebo-associated cancers, and were more likely to be lymph node positive, although this was of borderline significance. In the oestrogen-only arm, HRT-associated cancers were also larger (3 mm average difference), but there was no difference in lymph node involvement, and tumours were more likely to be lower grade (ie grade I/II) than were placebo-associated cancers. Based on the WHI study data, the estimated 10-year survival difference is very small (ie 1.5%) and probably accounts for an extra 1.4 breast cancer deaths per 1000 women in the age group 50–59 years with a history of exposure of combined HRT for 5 years immediately prior to diagnosis. There is no difference in the estimated survival comparing oestrogen alone associated with placebo-associated cancers based on the WHI data.

Breast cancer incidence and HRT use

Breast cancer incidence has been falling in countries such as the USA and Australia, and this has been attributed to declining HRT use since publication of the WHI studies. However, declining HRT use and reduction in breast cancer incidence do not necessarily establish a causal connection between the two. Moreover, the fall in the USA started in 1998, predating the first WHI publication. No such fall has been found in other countries such as the UK.

Endometrial cancer

Unopposed systemic oestrogen replacement therapy increases endometrial cancer risk. Most studies have shown that this excess risk is not completely eliminated with monthly sequential progestogen addition, especially when continued for more than 5 years. This has also been found with long-cycle HRT. No increased risk of endometrial cancer has been found with continuous combined regimens. Very low doses of systemic oestrogen (0.014 mg/day transdermal oestradiol patch) do not seem to stimulate the endometrium, but studies are limited and require confirmation. The increased risk of endometrial cancer with systemic oestrogen is lower than that found in obese or diabetic women.

Furthermore, oral but not vaginal treatment with low-potency formulations (such as oestriol) increases the RR of endometrial neoplasia.

Venous thromboembolism

Hormone replacement therapy increases the risk of venous thromboembolism (VTE) twofold, with the highest risk occurring in the first year of use. However, the absolute risk is small, being 1.7 per 1000 in women over 50 not taking HRT. Advancing age, obesity and an underlying thrombophilia risk factor, such as factor V Leiden, significantly increase the risk. Randomized trial data strongly suggest that women who have previously suffered VTE have an increased risk of recurrence in the first year of HRT use. Transdermal HRT may be associated with a lower risk even in women with thrombophilia. There may also be differences in progestogens, in that norpregnane derivatives may be thrombogenic, whereas micronized progesterone and pregnane derivatives do not increase risk.

Gallbladder disease

The WHI confirmed the observation of the Heart and Oestrogen/Progestin Replacement Study published in 1998 that HRT increases the risk of gallbladder disease. The MWS found that transdermal therapy entails a lower risk than oral. Gallbladder disease increases with ageing and with obesity, and, as a confounder, HRT users may have silent pre-existing disease.

Uncertainties

Cardiovascular disease (coronary heart disease and stroke)

The role of HRT in either primary or secondary prevention remains uncertain and currently should not be used primarily for this indication. Further investigation is still needed.

Coronary heart disease primary prevention

Until the late 1990s, oestrogen was thought to protect against coronary heart disease (CHD). Many cohort studies showed that HRT was associated with a 40–50% reduction in the incidence of CHD. The effects were the same for both oestrogen alone and combined HRT. However, the randomized, controlled WHI trial did not confirm the findings of the observational studies. Now it has become apparent that there are differences between HRT regimens, and that the timing of initiating HRT use may be crucial.

Combined versus oestrogen alone HRT

The WHI found an early, albeit transient, increase in coronary events in the combined but not the oestrogen-alone arm. Overall, there was no significant effect of HRT. The excess absolute risk at 50–59 years was 5; at 60–69 years, 1; and at 70–79 years, there were 23 cases of non-fatal myocardial infarction and death due to CHD per 10,000 women per year. In women within 10 years of menopause onset, there were four fewer cases than in controls. The WHI used medroxyprogesterone acetate as the progestogen, and there is little information about other progestogens that may have different effects on lipids, glucose, insulin metabolism and coagulation.

Analysis of the WHI oestrogen-alone study showed a non-significant reduction in CHD that was most marked in the younger (50–59 years) age group. In this subgroup, there was a significant reduction in a composite of coronary events and procedures, and there were no significant increases in events in the older age groups. The reduced absolute risk at 50–59 years was 10, and at 60–69 years, 5, with an excess risk of four cases in those aged 70–79 years per 10,000 women per year. In women within 10 years of the menopause onset, there were 14 fewer cases than in controls.

Oral versus transdermal therapy

Whether or not transdermal is better than oral delivery on CHD risk is uncertain but this is supported by observational studies showing a lower risk with the transdermal route.

Oestrogen dose

A possible explanation for early cardiovascular harm in the WHI study is an increase in thrombogenesis or abnormal cardiovascular remodelling. Both of these effects are dose dependent. Thus, although oestrogen has the potential to cause vascular benefit (as shown in observational and animal studies), high doses have the potential to cause vascular harm. The results combining the two arms of WHI are consistent with this hypothesis: reduced risk was found in women aged 50–69 years and increased risk in older women. Thus, the dose of oestrogen used in WHI may have been inappropriately high for older women and does not reflect European practice, where dose is usually decreased with increasing age.

Timing of treatment

Women in the WHI who started combined HRT within 10 years of the menopause had a lower risk of CHD than women who started later. Combining the two HRT arms showed that women who initiated hormone therapy closer to menopause tended to have reduced CHD risk in contrast to the increase in CHD risk among women more distant from the menopause.

The estimated absolute excess risk of CHD for women within 10 years of menopause was −6 per 10,000 person-years; for women 10–19 years since menopause began, +4 per 10,000 person-years; and for women 20 or more years from menopause onset, +16 per 10,000 person-years. For the age group of 50–59 years, the absolute excess risk was −2 per 10,000 person-years; for 60–69 years, −1 per 10,000 person-years; and for 70–79 years, +19 per 10,000 person-years. Furthermore, in the observational Nurses' Health Study, women beginning HRT near menopause had a significantly reduced risk of CHD (RR = 0.66, 95% CI 0.54–0.80 for oestrogen alone; RR = 0.72, 95% CI 0.56–0.92 for oestrogen with progestogen).

A *post hoc* WHI substudy in hysterectomized women aged below 60 years compared calcified plaque in the coronary arteries, a marker for atheromatous-plaque burden, which is predictive of future risk of cardiovascular events. Mean coronary-artery calcium score after trial completion was lower among women receiving oestrogen than among those receiving placebo. However, there were no baseline measurements and no measurements carried out in other age groups, so the value of these data is limited. A biological mechanism involving 27-hydroxycholesterol (27HC) has been postulated to explain why women in the WHI study who started HRT within 10 years of the menopause had a lower risk of CHD than women who started later. This cholesterol metabolite is elevated in hypercholesterolaemia, is found in atherosclerotic lesions, and is a competitive antagonist of oestrogen receptor action in the vasculature. The increasing presence of 27HC may be a contributing factor in the loss of oestrogen protection from vascular disease in older women. However, even in older women with established CHD, oestrogen has been shown to have certain beneficial arterial effects.

Premature menopause

Women with untreated premature menopause are at increased risk of CHD. Regulatory bodies recommend the use of HRT in premature ovarian failure up until the average age of the natural menopause.

Coronary heart disease secondary prevention

Although angiographic and cohort studies such as the Nurses' Health Study suggested a role of oestrogen in the secondary prevention of CHD, this has not been confirmed in randomized, controlled trials with both oral and transdermal therapy (Table 7.2).

Table 7.2

Randomized, controlled trials of hormone replacement therapy as secondary prevention for coronary heart disease

Study	Hormone replacement therapy	Route of administration	Relative risk (95% confidence interval) of acute myocardial infarction	Sample size
HERS (Hulley, 1998)	CEE/MPA	Oral	0.99 (0.8–1.22)	2769
PHASE (Clarke, 2002)	17β-oestradiol	Transdermal	1.29 (0.84–1.95)	255
WEST (Viscoli, 2001)	17β-oestradiol	Oral	1.1 (0.6–1.9)	664
ESPRIT (Cherry, 2002)	Oestradiol valerate	Oral	0.99 (0.7–1.41)	1017

CEE: conjugated equine oestrogens; MPA: medroxyprogesterone acetate

Stroke

Various observational data are available on HRT and stroke, but interpretation is difficult because of differences in study design and failure to distinguish between ischaemic and haemorrhagic stroke. Both arms of the WHI found an increase in ischaemic but not haemorrhagic stroke. However, age or time since menopause did not affect the risk of stroke in the WHI study. Moreover, in women who have experienced a previous ischaemic stroke, oestrogen replacement does not reduce mortality or recurrence as evidenced by randomized, controlled trials.

Dementia and cognition

While oestrogen may delay or reduce the risk of Alzheimer's disease (AD), it does not seem to improve established disease. It is unclear whether there is a critical age or duration of treatment for exposure to oestrogen to have an effect in prevention, but there may be a window of opportunity in the early postmenopause when the pathological processes that lead to AD (and CVD) are being initiated and when HRT may have a preventive effect. The WHI found a twofold increased risk of dementia in women with both oestrogen and progestogen and oestrogen alone. However, this increased risk was only significant in the group of women over the age of 75 years. Similarly, the WHI found deterioration in cognitive function in women aged over 65, especially in those with lower cognitive function at the initiation of treatment. It is not clear why these results are the opposite of earlier findings from observational studies and animal models. Current advances in scanning technology have observed a direct effect of oestrogen on cognitive function. More evidence is required, especially from younger postmenopausal women taking appropriate doses and different regimens, before definitive advice can be given in relation to dementia and cognition.

Ovarian cancer

On ovarian cancer, most data pertain to replacement with oestrogen alone with increasing risk in the very long term (>10 years). However, with continuous combined therapy, this increase does not seem apparent. This issue is unresolved and requires further examination, and there is currently insufficient evidence to recommend alterations in HRT prescribing practice.

Quality of life

While some studies have shown improvement in both symptomatic and asymptomatic women, others have not. This lack of effect seen in the WHI is hardly surprising, since the study participants were largely asymptomatic. This area is difficult to evaluate because of the different measures used, varying levels of menopausal symptomatology, a large placebo effect and extrinsic factors which may alter women's responses.

Tibolone

Tibolone is effective in treating menopausal symptoms. It conserves bone mass and reduces the risk of vertebral and non-vertebral fractures particularly in patients who had already had a vertebral fracture. It also reduces the risk of invasive breast cancer and colon cancer, but it does not significantly reduce the risk of hip fracture, and it increases the risk of stroke. However, it should be noted that, for the age group (60–85 years) included in the LIFT study, the incidence of stroke in the placebo group was 47% lower than that seen in other studies such as the WHI, for reasons unknown. Thus, the findings may reflect a decreased incidence of stroke in the placebo group more than an increased incidence in the tibolone group. The LIFT study also showed that it does not have a deleterious effect on CHD or VTE. The MWS showed an increased risk of breast cancer and endometrial cancer. However, the increased risk of endometrial cancer has not been confirmed in randomized, controlled trials. The LIBERATE randomized trial of tibolone in breast cancer survivors was discontinued early in 2007, as there was an excess of breast cancer recurrences in the group of women randomized to receive tibolone. As with HRT, one would suggest caution in initiating therapy with tibolone in women aged above 60 years.

Further reading

General

Heiss G, Wallace R, Anderson GL, *et al.* Health risks and benefits 3 years after stopping randomized treatment with estrogen and progestin. *JAMA* 2008;**299**: 1036–45.

Prentice RL, Anderson GL. The Women's Health Initiative: lessons learned. *Annu Rev Public Health* 2007;**29**:131–50.

Shapiro S. Recent epidemiological evidence relevant to the clinical management of the menopause. *Climacteric* 2007;**10**(Suppl 2):2–15.

Whitehead M, Farmer R. The Million Women Study: a critique. *Endocrine* 2004;**24**: 187–93.

Wittes J, Barrett-Connor E, Braunwald E, *et al.* Monitoring the randomized trials of the Women's Health Initiative: the experience of the Data and Safety Monitoring Board. *Clin Trials* 2007;**4**:218–34.

Vasomotor symptoms

Barnabei VM, Cochrane BB, Aragaki AK, *et al.* Menopausal symptoms and treatment-related effects of estrogen and progestin in the Women's Health Initiative. *Obstet Gynecol* 2005;**105**:1063–73.

MacLennan A, Lester S, Moore V. Oral oestrogen replacement therapy versus placebo for hot flushes. *Cochrane Database Syst Rev* 2001;**1**:CD002978.

Simon JA, Snabes MC. Menopausal hormone therapy for vasomotor symptoms: balancing the risks and benefits with ultra-low doses of estrogen. *Expert Opin Investig Drugs* 2007;**16**:2005–20.

Urogenital symptoms and sexuality

Cardozo L, Bachmann G, McClish D, *et al.* Meta-analysis of estrogen therapy in the management of urogenital atrophy in postmenopausal women: second report of the Hormones and Urogenital Therapy Committee. *Obstet Gynecol* 1998;**92**: 722–7.

Kingsberg S. Testosterone treatment for hypoactive sexual desire disorder in postmenopausal women. *J Sex Med* 2007;**4**(Suppl 3):227–34.

Perrotta C, Aznar M, Mejia R, *et al.* Oestrogens for preventing recurrent urinary tract infection in postmenopausal women. *Cochrane Database Syst Rev* 2008;**2**: CD005131.

Rozenberg S, Pastijn A, Gevers R, Murillo D. Estrogen therapy in older patients with recurrent urinary tract infections: a review. *Int J Fertil Womens Med* 2004;**49**: 71–4.

Tomlinson J, Rees M, Mander T, eds. *Sexual Health and the Menopause*. London: RSM Press, 2005.

Osteoporosis

Bagger YZ, Tankó LB, Alexandersen P, *et al.* Two to three years of hormone replacement treatment in healthy women have long-term preventive effects on bone mass and osteoporotic fractures: the PERF study. *Bone* 2004;**34**:728–35.

Cauley JA, Robbins J, Chen Z, *et al.*; for the Women's Health Initiative Investigators. Effects of estrogen plus progestin on risk of fracture and bone mineral density: the Women's Health Initiative Randomized Trial. *JAMA* 2003;**290**:1729–38.

Ettinger B, Ensrud KE, Wallace R, *et al.* Effects of ultralow-dose transdermal estradiol on bone mineral density: a randomized clinical trial. *Obstet Gynecol* 2004;**104**: 443–51.

Medicines and Healthcare Products Regulatory Agency and Commission on Human Medicines. Hormone replacement therapy: updated advice. *Drug Safety Update* 2007;**1**: 2–5.

North American Menopause Society. Management of osteoporosis in postmenopausal women: 2006 position statement of the North American Menopause Society. *Menopause* 2006;**13**:340–67.

Stevenson JC and on behalf of the International Consensus Group on HRT and Regulatory Issues. HRT, osteoporosis and regulatory authorities. *Quis custodiet ipsos custodes? Hum Reprod* 2006;**21**:1668–71.

Women's Health Initiative Steering Committee. Effects of conjugated equine estrogen in postmenopausal women with hysterectomy: the Women's Health Initiative Randomized Controlled Trial. *JAMA* 2004;**291**:1701–12.

Writing Group on Osteoporosis for the British Menopause Society Council; Al-Azzawi F, Barlow D, Hillard T, *et al.* Prevention and treatment of osteoporosis in women. *Menopause Int* 2007;**13**:178–81.

Colorectal cancer

Corrao G, Zambon A, Conti V, *et al.* Menopause hormone replacement therapy and cancer risk: an Italian record linkage investigation. *Ann Oncol* 2008;**19**:150–5.

Murff HJ, Shrubsole MJ, Smalley WE, *et al.* The interaction of age and hormone replacement therapy on colon adenoma risk. *Cancer Detect Prev* 2007;**31**:161–5.

Women's Health Initiative Steering Committee. Effects of conjugated equine estrogen in postmenopausal women with hysterectomy: the Women's Health Initiative Randomized Controlled Trial. *JAMA* 2004;**291**:1701–12.

Writing Group for the Women's Health Initiative Investigators. Risks and benefits of estrogen plus progestin in healthy postmenopausal women: principal results from the Women's Health Initiative Randomized Controlled Trial. *JAMA* 2002;**288**:321–33.

Breast cancer

American Cancer Society. Breast cancer facts and figures 2007–2008. www.cancer.org/downloads/STT/BCFF-Final.pdf.

Anderson GL, Chlebowski RT, Rossouw JE, *et al.*; Cancer Research UK. UK breast cancer incidence statistics. info.cancerresearchuk.org/cancerstats/types/breast/incidence/.

Canfell K, Banks E, Moa AM, Beral V. Decrease in breast cancer incidence following a rapid fall in use of hormone replacement therapy in Australia. *Med J Aust* 2008;**188**:641–4.

Chlebowski RT, Hendrix SL, Langer RD, *et al*. Influence of estrogen plus progestin on breast cancer and mammography in healthy postmenopausal women. The Women's Health Initiative Randomized Trial. *JAMA* 2003;**289**:3243–53.

Collaborative Group on Hormonal Factors in Breast Cancer. Breast cancer and hormone replacement therapy: collaborative reanalysis of data from 51 epidemiological studies of 52,705 women with breast cancer and 108,411 women without breast cancer. *Lancet* 1997;**350**:1047–59.

Collins JA, Blake JM, Crosignani PG. Breast cancer risk with postmenopausal hormonal treatment. *Hum Reprod Update* 2005;**11**:545–60.

Ewertz M, Mellemkjaer L, Poulsen AH, *et al*. Hormone use for menopausal symptoms and risk of breast cancer. A Danish cohort study. *Br J Cancer* 2005;**92**:1293–7.

Li CI, Daling JR. Changes in breast cancer incidence rates in the United States by histologic subtype and race/ethnicity, 1995 to 2004. *Cancer Epidemiol Biomarkers Prev* 2007;**16**:2773–80.

Li CI, Malone KE, Porter PL, *et al*. Relationship between menopausal hormone therapy and risk of ductal, lobular, and ductal-lobular breast carcinomas. *Cancer Epidemiol Biomarkers Prev* 2008;**17**:43–50.

Million Women Study Collaborators. The Million Women Study: design and characteristics of the study population. *Breast Cancer Res* 1999;**1**:73–80.

Million Women Study Collaborators. Breast cancer and hormone-replacement therapy in the Million Women Study. *Lancet* 2003;**362**:419–27.

Reeves GK, Pirie K, Beral V, *et al*.; Million Women Study Collaboration. Cancer incidence and mortality in relation to body mass index in the Million Women Study: cohort study. *BMJ* 2007;**335**(7630):1134.

Ritenbaugh C. Prior hormone therapy and breast cancer risk in the Women's Health Initiative randomized trial of estrogen plus progestin. *Maturitas* 2006;**55**:103–15.

Stefanick ML, Anderson GL, Margolis KL, *et al*. Effects of conjugated equine estrogens on breast cancer and mammography screening in postmenopausal women with hysterectomy. *JAMA* 2006;**295**:1647–57.

Women's Health Initiative Steering Committee. Effects of conjugated equine estrogen in postmenopausal women with hysterectomy: the Women's Health Initiative Randomized Controlled Trial. *JAMA* 2004;**291**:1701–12.

Endometrial cancer

Anderson GL, Judd HL, Kaunitz AM, *et al*.; Women's Health Initiative Investigators. Effects of estrogen plus progestin on gynecologic cancers and associated diagnostic procedures: the Women's Health Initiative Randomized Trial. *JAMA* 2003;**290**: 1739–48.

Beral V, Bull D, Reeves G; Million Women Study Collaborators. Endometrial cancer and hormone-replacement therapy in the Million Women Study. *Lancet* 2005;**365**: 1543–51.

Diem S, Grady D, Quan J, *et al.* Effects of ultralow-dose transdermal estradiol on postmenopausal symptoms in women aged 60 to 80 years. *Menopause* 2006;**13**: 130–8.

Erkkola R, Kumento U, Lehmuskoski S, *et al.* No increased risk of endometrial hyperplasia with fixed long-cycle oestrogen-progestogen therapy after five years. *J Br Menopause Soc* 2004;**10**:9–13.

Johnson SR, Ettinger B, Macer JL, *et al.* Uterine and vaginal effects of unopposed ultralow-dose transdermal estradiol. *Obstet Gynecol* 2005;**105**:779–87.

Lacey JV Jr, Leitzmann MF, Chang SC, *et al.* Endometrial cancer and menopausal hormone therapy in the National Institutes of Health-AARP Diet and Health Study cohort. *Cancer* 2007;**109**:1303–11.

McCullough ML, Patel AV, Patel R, *et al.* Body mass and endometrial cancer risk by hormone replacement therapy and cancer subtype. *Cancer Epidemiol Biomarkers Prev* 2008;**17**:73–9.

Pukkala E, Tulenheimo-Silfvast A, Leminen A. Incidence of cancer among women using long versus monthly cycle hormonal replacement therapy, Finland 1994–1997. *Cancer Causes Control* 2001;**12**:111–15.

Reeves GK, Pirie K, Beral V, *et al.*; Million Women Study Collaboration. Cancer incidence and mortality in relation to body mass index in the Million Women Study: cohort study. *BMJ* 2007;**335**:1134.

Weiderpass E, Adami HO, Baron JA, *et al.* Risk of endometrial cancer following estrogen replacement with and without progestins. *J Natl Cancer Inst* 1999;**91**:1131–7.

Weiderpass E, Baron JA, Adami HO, *et al.* Low-potency oestrogen and risk of endometrial cancer: a case-control study. *Lancet* 1999;**353**:1824–8.

Weiderpass E, Persson I, Adami HO, *et al.* Body size in different periods of life, diabetes mellitus, hypertension, and risk of postmenopausal endometrial cancer (Sweden). *Cancer Causes Control* 2000;**11**:185–92.

Venous thromboembolism

Canonico M, Oger E, Plu-Bureau G, *et al.*; Estrogen and Thromboembolism Risk (ESTHER) Study Group. Hormone therapy and venous thromboembolism among postmenopausal women: impact of the route of estrogen administration and progestogens: the ESTHER study. *Circulation* 2007;**115**:840–5.

Canonico M, Plu-Bureau G, Lowe GD, Scarabin PY. Hormone replacement therapy and risk of venous thromboembolism in postmenopausal women: systematic review and meta-analysis. *BMJ* 2008;**336**:1227–31.

Curb JD, Prentice RL, Bray PF, *et al.* Venous thrombosis and conjugated equine estrogen in women without a uterus. *Arch Intern Med* 2006;**166**:772–80.

Cushman M, Kuller LH, Prentice R, *et al.*; Women's Health Initiative Investigators. Estrogen plus progestin and risk of venous thrombosis. *JAMA* 2004;**292**:1573–80.

Hoibraaten E, Qvigstad E, Arnesen H, *et al.* Increased risk of recurrent venous thromboembolism during hormone replacement therapy – results of the randomized, double-blind, placebo-controlled estrogen in venous thromboembolism trial (EVTET). *Thromb Haemost* 2000;**84**:961–7.

Straczek C, Oger E, Yon de Jonage-Canonico MB, *et al.*; Estrogen and Thromboembolism Risk (ESTHER) Study Group. Prothrombotic mutations, hormone therapy, and venous thromboembolism among postmenopausal women: impact of the route of estrogen administration. *Circulation* 2005;**112**:3495–3500.

Gallbladder disease

Cirillo DJ, Wallace RB, Rodabough RJ, *et al.* Effect of estrogen therapy on gallbladder disease. *JAMA* 2005;**293**:330–9.

Hulley S, Grady D, Bush T, *et al.* Randomized trial of estrogen plus progestin for secondary prevention of coronary heart disease in postmenopausal women. Heart and Estrogen/Progestin Replacement Study (HERS) Research Group. *JAMA* 1998;**280**:605–13.

Liu B, Beral V, Balkwill A, *et al.* for the Million Women Study Collaborators. Gallbladder disease and use of transdermal versus oral hormone replacement therapy in postmenopausal women: prospective cohort study. *BMJ* 2008;**337**: a386.

Portincasa P, Moschetta A, Petruzzelli M, *et al.* Gallstone disease: symptoms and diagnosis of gallbladder stones. *Best Pract Res Clin Gastroenterol* 2006;**20**:1017–29.

Cardiovascular disease (coronary heart disease and stroke)

Billeci AM, Paciaroni M, Caso V, Agnelli G. Hormone replacement therapy and stroke. *Curr Vasc Pharmacol* 2008;**6**:112–23.

Cherry N, Gilmour K, Hannaford P, *et al.* Oestrogen therapy for prevention of reinfarction in postmenopausal women: a randomised placebo controlled trial. *Lancet* 2002;**360**:2001–8.

Clarke SC, Kelleher J, Lloyd-Jones H, *et al.* A study of hormone replacement therapy in postmenopausal women with ischaemic heart disease: the Papworth HRT atherosclerosis study. *Br J Obstet Gynaecol* 2002;**109**:1056–62.

Collins P, Flather M, Lees B, *et al.* (Women's Hormone Intervention Secondary Prevention Study); Pilot Study Investigators. Randomized trial of effects of continuous combined HRT on markers of lipids and coagulation in women with acute coronary syndromes: WHISP Pilot Study. *Eur Heart J* 2006;**27**:2046–53.

Collins P, Rosano GM, Sarrel PM, *et al.* 17[beta]-Estradiol attenuates acetylcholine-induced coronary arterial constriction in women but not men with coronary heart disease. *Circulation* 1995;**92**:24–30.

Grady D, Herrington D, Bittner V, *et al.*; HERS Research Group. Cardiovascular disease outcomes during 6.8 years of hormone therapy: Heart and Estrogen/Progestin Replacement Study follow-up (HERS II). *JAMA* 2002;**288**:49–57.

Grodstein F, Manson JE, Stampfer MJ. Postmenopausal hormone use and secondary prevention of coronary events in the Nurses' Health Study. a prospective, observational study. *Ann Intern Med* 2001;**135**:1–8.

Grodstein F, Manson JE, Stampfer MJ. Hormone therapy and coronary heart disease: the role of time since menopause and age at hormone initiation. *J Womens Health* 2006;**15**:35–44.

Hsia J, Langer RD, Manson JE, *et al.* Conjugated equine estrogens and coronary heart disease. *Arch Intern Med* 2006;**166**:357–65.

Hulley S, Grady D, Bush T, *et al.* Randomized trial of estrogen plus progestin for secondary prevention of coronary heart disease in postmenopausal women. Heart and Estrogen/Progestin Replacement Study (HERS) Research Group. *JAMA* 1998;**280**:605–13.

Lobo RA. Surgical menopause and cardiovascular risks. *Menopause* 2007;**14**: 562–6.

Løkkegaard E, Andreasen AH, Jacobsen RK, *et al.* Hormone therapy and risk of myocardial infarction: a national register study. *Eur Heart J* 2008;**29**:2660–8.

Løkkegaard E, Jovanovic Z, Heitmann BL, *et al.* The association between early menopause and risk of ischaemic heart disease: influence of hormone therapy. *Maturitas* 2006;**53**:226–33.

Manson JE, Allison MA, Rossouw JE, *et al.*; WHI and WHI-CACS Investigators. Estrogen therapy and coronary-artery calcification. *N Engl J Med* 2007;**356**: 2591–2602.

Manson JE, Hsia J, Johnson KC, *et al.*; Women's Health Initiative Investigators. Estrogen plus progestin and the risk of coronary heart disease. *N Engl J Med* 2003;**349**:523–34.

Prentice RL, Langer RD, Stefanick ML, *et al.* Combined analysis of Women's Health Initiative observational and clinical trial data on postmenopausal hormone treatment and cardiovascular disease. *Am J Epidemiol* 2006;**163**:589–99.

Rossouw JE, Anderson GL, Prentice RL. Risks and benefits of estrogen plus progestin in healthy postmenopausal women: principal results from the Women's Health Initiative Randomized Controlled Trial. *JAMA* 2002;**288**:321–33.

Rossouw JE, Prentice RL, Manson JE, *et al.* Postmenopausal hormone therapy and risk of cardiovascular disease by age and years since menopause. *JAMA* 2007;**297**: 1465–77.

Stevenson JC. HRT and the primary prevention of cardiovascular disease. *Maturitas* 2007;**57**:31–4.

Women's Health Initiative Steering Committee. Effects of conjugated equine estrogen in postmenopausal women with hysterectomy: the Women's Health Initiative Randomized Controlled Trial. *JAMA* 2004;**291**:1701–12.

Umetani M, Domoto H, Gormley AK, *et al.* 27-Hydroxycholesterol is an endogenous SERM that inhibits the cardiovascular effects of estrogen. *Nat Med* 2007;**13**: 1185–92.

Viscoli CM, Brass LM, Kernan WN, *et al.* A clinical trial of estrogen-replacement therapy after ischemic stroke. *N Engl J Med* 2001;**345**:1243–9.

Dementia and cognition

Barber B, Daley S, O'Brien J. Dementia. In: Keith L, Rees M, Mander T, eds. *Menopause, Postmenopause and Ageing.* London: RSM Press, 2005:20–34.

Espeland MA, Rapp SR, Shumaker SA, *et al.* Conjugated equine estrogens and global cognitive function in postmenopausal women: Women's Health Initiative Memory Study. *JAMA* 2004;**291**:2959–68.

Rapp SR, Espeland MA, Shumaker SA, *et al.* Effect of estrogen plus progestin on global cognitive function in postmenopausal women: the Women's Health Initiative Memory Study: a randomized controlled trial. *JAMA* 2003;**289**:2663–72.

Rasgon NL, Magnusson C, Johansen AL, *et al.* Endogenous and exogenous hormone exposure and risk of cognitive impairment in Swedish twins: a preliminary study. *Psychoneuroendocrinology* 2005;**30**:558–67.

Shaywitz SE, Shaywitz BA, Pugh KR, *et al.* Effect of estrogen on brain activation patterns in postmenopausal women during working memory tasks. *JAMA* 1999;**281**:1197–1202.

Shumaker SA, Legault C, Kuller L, *et al.* Conjugated equine estrogens and incidence of probable dementia and mild cognitive impairment in postmenopausal women: Women's Health Initiative Memory Study. *JAMA* 2004;**291**:2947–58.

Shumaker SA, Legault C, Rapp SR, *et al.* Estrogen plus progestin and the incidence of dementia and mild cognitive impairment in postmenopausal women: the Women's Health Initiative Memory Study: a randomized controlled trial. *JAMA* 2003;**289**:2651–62.

Ovarian cancer

Anderson GL, Judd HL, Kaunitz AM, *et al.*; Women's Health Initiative Investigators. Effects of estrogen plus progestin on gynecologic cancers and associated diagnostic procedures: the Women's Health Initiative Randomized Trial. *JAMA* 2003;**290**: 1739–48.

Beral V; Million Women Study Collaborators, Bull D, Green J, Reeves G. Ovarian cancer and hormone replacement therapy in the Million Women Study. *Lancet* 2007;**369**:1703–10.

Danforth KN, Tworoger SS, Hecht JL, *et al.* A prospective study of postmenopausal hormone use and ovarian cancer risk. *Br J Cancer* 2007;**96**:151–6.

Lacey JV Jr, Brinton LA, Leitzmann MF, *et al.* Menopausal hormone therapy and ovarian cancer risk in the National Institutes of Health-AARP Diet and Health Study Cohort. *J Natl Cancer Inst* 2006;**98**:1397–1405.

Quality of life

Hays J, Ockene JK, Brunner RL, *et al.* Effects of estrogen plus progestin on health-related quality of life. *N Engl J Med* 2003;**348**:1839–54.

Pitkin J, Smetnik VP, Vadász P, *et al.*; Indivina 321 Study Group. Continuous combined hormone replacement therapy relieves climacteric symptoms and improves health-related quality of life in early postmenopausal women. *Menopause Int* 2007;**13**:116–23.

Welton AJ, Vickers MR, Kim J, *et al.*; WISDOM team. Health related quality of life after combined hormone replacement therapy: randomised controlled trial. *BMJ* 2008;**337**:a1190.

Ylikangas S, Sintonen H, Heikkinen J. Decade-long use of continuous combined hormone replacement therapy is associated with better health-related quality of life in postmenopausal women, as measured by the generic 15D instrument. *J Br Menopause Soc* 2005;**11**:145–51.

Tibolone

Archer DF, Hendrix S, Ferenczy A, *et al.*; THEBES Study Group. Tibolone histology of the endometrium and breast endpoints study: design of the trial and endometrial histology at baseline in postmenopausal women. *Fertil Steril* 2007;**88**:866–78.

Archer DF, Hendrix S, Gallagher JC, *et al.* Endometrial effects of tibolone. *J Clin Endocrinol Metab* 2007;**92**:911–18.

Beral V, Bull D, Reeves G; Million Women Study Collaborators. Endometrial cancer and hormone-replacement therapy in the Million Women Study. *Lancet* 2005;**365**: 1543–51.

Cummings SR, Ettinger B, Delmas PD, *et al.* The effects of tibolone in older post-menopausal women. *N Engl J Med* 2008;**359**:697–708.

Ettinger B, Kenemans P, Johnson SR, *et al.* Endometrial effects of tibolone in elderly, osteoporotic women. *Obstet Gynecol* 2008;**112**:653–9.

Million Women Study Collaborators. Breast cancer and hormone-replacement therapy in the Million Women Study. *Lancet* 2003;**362**:419–27.

Opatrny L, Dell'Aniello S, Assouline S, Suissa S. Hormone replacement therapy use and variations in the risk of breast cancer. *BJOG* 2008;**115**:169–75.

Swegle JM, Kelly MW. Tibolone: a unique version of hormone replacement therapy. *Ann Pharmacother* 2004;**38**:874–81.

8 Non-oestrogen-based treatments for menopausal symptoms

Hot flushes
Urogenital problems
Lack of sexual desire
Further reading

Non-oestrogen-based treatments are used to treat hot flushes, symptoms of urogenital atrophy and lack of sexual desire. Non-hormonal and hormonal strategies will be discussed.

Hot flushes

Hot flushes are the most common menopausal symptoms and may last for several years. Concerns about the adverse effects of oestrogen have led to increased interest in other therapies. Several have been studied.

Clonidine

Clonidine is a centrally acting alpha-adrenoceptor agonist that was developed originally for the treatment of hypertension. While it has been one of the most popular non-hormonal preparations for the treatment of vasomotor symptoms since the early 1980s, the evidence for efficacy is conflicting in randomized, controlled trials. However, it may be of limited help in women with tamoxifen-induced hot flushes. Clonidine is the only non-oestrogen-based preparation licensed for menopausal flushing. Side-effects include dry mouth, sedation, dizziness, nausea and nocturnal restlessness. The dose is 50–75 µg twice daily.

Selective serotonin reuptake inhibitors and serotonin and noradrenaline reuptake inhibitors

The selective serotonin reuptake inhibitors (SSRIs) fluoxetine, paroxetine, citalopram and venlafaxine have been found to be effective in several studies. However, most are short-lasting, effective for only a few weeks. A 9-month, placebo-controlled study of the SSRIs citalopram and fluoxetine showed no benefit. Side-effects include gastrointestinal symptoms (nausea) and sexual dysfunction (delayed or absent orgasm). Some early evidence suggests that SSRIs may cause bone loss. The most convincing data for improvement of hot flushes are for the serotonin and noradrenaline reuptake inhibitor SNRI venlafaxine at a dose of 37.5 mg bd. A randomized trial of a new SNRI, desvenlafaxine, has shown a 64% reduction of hot flushes at 12 weeks.

Gabapentin

Gabapentin is a gamma-aminobutyric acid analogue used to treat epilepsy, neurogenic pain and migraine. It reduces hot flushes at a dose of 900 mg/day by about 50%. The side-effects of dry mouth, dizziness and drowsiness may improve with continued use.

Progestogens

Progestogens such as 5 mg/day norethisterone or 40 mg/day megestrol acetate can be effective in controlling hot flushes and night sweats. The availability of megestrol acetate 40 mg tablets varies worldwide. Of concern, with doses of progestogens that achieve control of vasomotor symptoms, the risk of venous thromboembolism may be increased. Safety with regard to the breast is also uncertain.

Other drugs

The antidepressants veralipride and moclobemide have also been studied. However, they are of limited effectiveness and there are concerns about adverse effects. Beta blockers were advocated in the early 1980s, but, again, the evidence is poor.

Urogenital problems

While many lubricants and vaginal moisturizers are available without prescription, two can be prescribed in the UK (Replens and Sylk). Lubricants usually consist of a combination of protectants and thickening agents in a water-soluble base. They are usually used to relieve vaginal dryness during intercourse. They therefore do not provide a long-term solution. Lubricants must be applied frequently for more continuous relief and require reapplication before intercourse.

Lubricants such as petroleum-based products and baby oil can compromise the integrity of condoms. This is important when condoms are used for contraception and/or to prevent sexually transmitted infections.

Moisturizers may contain a bioadhesive polycarbophil-based polymer, which attaches to mucin and epithelial cells on the vaginal wall and retains water. Moisturizers are promoted as providing long-term relief of vaginal dryness and need to be applied less frequently.

Lack of sexual desire

This is a common problem, affecting around 40% of postmenopausal women. Management plans can be divided into non-hormonal and hormonal. They can be used together. Psychosexual therapy (or psychosexual counselling) has proven success rates. Both partners should be encouraged to attend. Following initial assessment, the therapist will give the couple information about how sexual problems arise and the various treatment options available. It is important to ensure that the sex therapist is qualified and abides by the codes of ethics of an appropriate professional body.

Several studies have shown the benefit of testosterone therapy in postmenopausal women but mainly in those using oestrogen. In the UK, the only licensed preparations for women for many years were subcutaneous implants or pellets to be put under the skin under local anaesthesia. Testosterone patches (300 µg) for women are now available. These have the advantage that women can start and stop treatment whenever they want. They are currently licensed for hysterectomized and oophorectomized women taking concomitant oestradiol-based hormone replacement therapy. However, they are also effective in naturally menopausal women taking oestrogen.

Tibolone is a synthetic steroid with oestrogenic, progestogenic and androgenic properties. Its therapeutic indication is the treatment of oestrogen-deficiency symptoms (including vasomotor symptoms, depressed mood, decreased libido) in postmenopausal women.

Further reading

Hot flushes

Butt DA, Lock M, Lewis JE, *et al.* Gabapentin for the treatment of menopausal hot flashes: a randomized controlled trial. *Menopause* 2008;**15**:310–18.

Diem SJ, Blackwell TL, Stone KL, *et al.* Use of antidepressants and rates of hip bone loss in older women: the study of osteoporotic fractures. *Arch Intern Med* 2007;**167**:1240–5.

Evans ML, Pritts E, Vittinghoff E, *et al.* Management of postmenopausal hot flushes with venlafaxine hydrochloride: a randomized, controlled trial. *Obstet Gynecol* 2005;**105**:161–6.

Guttuso T Jr, Kurlan R, McDermott MP, Kieburz K. Gabapentin's effects on hot flashes in postmenopausal women: a randomized controlled trial. *Obstet Gynecol* 2003;**101**:337–45.

Liang Y, Besch-Williford C, Brekken RA, Hyder SM. Progestin-dependent progression of human breast tumor xenografts: a novel model for evaluating antitumor therapeutics. *Cancer Res* 2007;**67**:9929–36.

Loprinzi CL, Kugler JW, Sloan JA, *et al*. Venlafaxine in the management of hot flashes in survivors of breast cancer: a randomised controlled trial. *Lancet* 2000;**356**: 2059–63.

Loprinzi CL, Michalak JC, Quella SK, *et al*. Megestrol acetate for the prevention of hot flashes. *N Engl J Med* 1994;**331**:347–52.

Loprinzi CL, Sloan JA, Perez EA, *et al*. Phase III evaluation of fluoxetine for treatment of hot flashes. *J Clin Oncol* 2002;**20**:1578–83.

Nelson HD, Vesco KK, Haney E, *et al*. Nonhormonal therapies for menopausal hot flashes: systematic review and meta-analysis. *JAMA* 2006;**295**:2057–71.

Pandya KJ, Morrow GR, Roscoe JA, *et al*. Gabapentin for hot flashes in 420 women with breast cancer: a double-blind placebo-controlled trial. *Lancet* 2005;**366**: 818–24.

Pandya KJ, Raubertas RF, Flynn PJ, *et al*. Oral clonidine in postmenopausal patients with breast cancer experiencing tamoxifen-induced hot flashes: a University of Rochester Cancer Center Community Clinical Oncology Program study. *Ann Intern Med* 2000;**132**:788–93.

Royal College and Obstetricians and Gynaecologists (RCOG). *Alternatives to HRT for the Management of Symptoms of the Menopause*. Scientific Advisory Committee Opinion Paper 6. London: RCOG, 2006. www.rcog.org.uk/index.asp? PageID=1561.

Speroff L, Gass M, Constantine G, Olivier S; Study 315 Investigators. Efficacy and tolerability of desvenlafaxine succinate treatment for menopausal vasomotor symptoms: a randomized controlled trial. *Obstet Gynecol* 2008;**111**:77–87.

Stearns V, Beebe KL, Iyengar M, Dube E. Paroxetine controlled release in the treatment of menopausal hot flashes: a randomised controlled trial. *JAMA* 2003;**289**: 2827–34.

Stimmel GL, Gutierrez MA. Sexual dysfunction and psychotropic medications. *CNS Spectr* 2006;**11**(Suppl 9):24–30.

Suvanto-Luukkonen E, Koivunen R, Sundstrom H, *et al*. Citalopram and fluoxetine in the treatment of postmenopausal symptoms: a prospective, randomized, 9-month, placebo-controlled, double-blind study. *Menopause* 2005;**12**:18–26.

Vasilakis C, Jick H, del Mar Melero-Montes M. Risk of idiopathic venous thromboembolism in users of progestagens alone. *Lancet* 1999;**354**:1610–11.

Wren BG, Brown LB. A double blind trial with clonidine and a placebo to treat hot flushes. *Med J Aust* 1986;**144**:369–70.

Urogenital problems

Bygdeman M, Swahn ML. Replens versus dienoestrol cream in the symptomatic treatment of vaginal atrophy in postmenopausal women. *Maturitas* 1996;**23**:259–63.

Castelo-Branco C, Cancelo MJ, Villero J, *et al*. Management of post-menopausal vaginal atrophy and atrophic vaginitis. *Maturitas* 2005;**52**(Suppl 1):S46–52.

Rosen AD, Rosen T. Study of condom integrity after brief exposure to over-the-counter vaginal preparations. *South Med J* 1999;**92**:305–7.

Lack of sexual desire

Braunstein GD, Sundwall DA, Katz M, *et al*. Safety and efficacy of a testosterone patch for the treatment of hypoactive sexual desire disorder in surgically menopausal women: a randomized, placebo-controlled trial. *Arch Intern Med* 2005;**165**: 1582–9.

Davis SR, Moreau M, Kroll R, *et al*; APHRODITE Study Team. Testosterone for low libido in postmenopausal women not taking estrogen. *N Engl J Med* 2008; **359**:2005–17.

Davis SR, van der Mooren MJ, van Lunsen RH, *et al*. Efficacy and safety of a testosterone patch for the treatment of hypoactive sexual desire disorder in surgically menopausal women: a randomized, placebo-controlled trial. *Menopause* 2006;**13**: 387–96.

Egarter C, Topcuoglu A, Vogl S, Sator M. Hormone replacement therapy with tibolone: effects on sexual functioning in postmenopausal women. *Acta Obstet Gynecol Scand* 2002;**81**:649–53.

Lindau ST, Schumm LP, Laumann EO, *et al*. A study of sexuality and health among older adults in the United States. *N Engl J Med* 2007;**357**:762–74.

Shifren JL, Davis SR, Moreau M, *et al*. Testosterone patch for the treatment of hypoactive sexual desire disorder in naturally menopausal women: results from the INTI-MATE NM1 Study. *Menopause* 2006;**13**:770–9.

Simon J, Braunstein G, Nachtigall L, *et al*. Testosterone patch increases sexual activity and desire in surgically menopausal women with hypoactive sexual desire disorder. *J Clin Endocrinol Metab* 2005;**90**:5226–33.

Tomlinson JM, Rees M, Mander T, eds. *Sexual Health and the Menopause*. London: RSM Press and British Menopause Society Publications, 2005.

Wylie KR. Sexuality and the menopause. *J Br Menopause Soc* 2006;**12**:149–52.

9 Non-oestrogen-based therapy for osteoporosis

> **Pharmacological interventions**
> **Non-pharmacological interventions**
> **Future developments**
> **Further reading**

The number of pharmacological and non-pharmacological interventions has expanded greatly over the past few years in response to the increasing concerns about the implications of osteoporosis in an ageing population.

Pharmacological interventions

All pharmacological interventions (Table 9.1) except for parathyroid hormone and strontium ranelate act mainly by inhibiting bone resorption. Very few data exist about long-term efficacy in reducing fractures (that is, more than 10 years of treatment) and safety of combinations of therapy. Comparative studies with fracture endpoints are limited. In many of the studies, the placebo group received calcium and vitamin D supplements.

Bisphosphonates

Bisphosphonates are chemical analogues of naturally occurring pyrophosphates thus allowing them to be integrated into the skeleton.

Bisphosphonates can be classified into two groups:

- non-nitrogen-containing bisphosphonates, such as etidronate
- nitrogen-containing bisphosphonates, such as alendronate, risedronate, ibandronate and zoledronic acid.

All bisphosphonates are absorbed poorly from the gastrointestinal tract and must be given on an empty stomach. Food or calcium-containing drinks (except water) inhibit the absorption, which at best is only 5–10% of the administered dose. The principal side-effect of all bisphosphonates is irritation of the upper gastrointestinal tract. Symptoms resolve quickly after drug withdrawal, and these adverse effects are much reduced by using weekly or monthly rather than daily regimens.

Table 9.1

Interventions for the prevention and treatment of osteoporosis

	Spine	Hip
Bisphosphonates		
Etidronate	A	B
Alendronate	A	A
Risedronate	A	A
Ibandronate	A	ND
Zoledronic acid	A	A
Calcium and Vitamin D	ND	A
Calcium	A	B
Calcitriol	A	ND
Calcitonin	A	B
Oestrogen	A	A
Raloxifene	A	ND
Strontium ranelate	A	A
Parathyroid hormone peptides	A	ND

ND: not demonstrated
The levels of evidence for the various agents detailed are as follows:
A = meta-analysis of randomized, controlled trials (RCTs) or from at least one
RCT/from at least one well-designed, controlled study without randomization;
B = from at least one other type of well-designed quasi-experimental study/from
well-designed non-experimental descriptive studies such as comparative studies,
correlation studies, or case-control studies

Their metabolism is an extremely slow process; indeed, the half-life of alendronate has been estimated to be as long as 12 years. There are concerns about effects on the fetal skeleton, and bisphosphonates are not advised in women with fertility aspirations.

Alendronate, risedronate, etidronate and ibandronate are used in the prevention and treatment of osteoporosis. The indication for zoledronic acid is the treatment of osteoporosis in postmenopausal women at increased risk of fracture. The first three are also used in corticosteroid-induced osteoporosis.

The question of how long to prescribe a bisphosphonate has not been fully clarified yet, because of concerns about 'frozen bone', with complete turning off of bone remodelling with long-term use and also development of osteonecrosis in the jaw. Five years of treatment with a 2-year 'holiday' has been proposed for alendronate, but differences may exist with individual bisphosphonates. This may not be applicable to glucocorticoid-induced osteoporosis.

The vast majority of reports of osteonecrosis refer to high-dose intra-venous bisphosphonates used in the oncological setting. Very few cases have been reported in women using oral bisphosphonates for osteoporosis. At this stage, clinical practice should not necessarily be altered, but dental review could be considered in women with significant dental disease.

There have been concerns about atrial fibrillation with bisphosphonates but mainly with intravenous regimens, and the mechanism is uncertain.

Comparisons have been made between alendronate and risedronate and between alendronate and raloxifene, but so far they have been mainly limited to their effects on bone mineral density (BMD) rather than the risk of fracture. Randomized, controlled trials (RCTs) are awaited.

Alendronate reduces vertebral and non-vertebral fractures by 50% in RCTs. The dose for prevention of osteoporosis is 5 mg/day or 35 mg once weekly; for the treatment of established disease, it is 10 mg/day or 70 mg once weekly.

Risedronate reduces vertebral and non-vertebral fractures in RCTs. The dose for treatment of established disease is 5 mg/day or 35 mg once weekly.

Ibandronate reduces vertebral but not non-vertebral fractures by 50% in RCTs undertaken in postmenopausal women. The dose is 2.5 mg/day or 150 mg once monthly, orally, or 3 mg intravenously every 3 months.

Etidronate reduces the risk of vertebral but not non-vertebral fractures. It is given intermittently (400 mg on 14 out of every 90 days) with 1250 mg of calcium carbonate (which when dissolved in water provides 500 mg of calcium as calcium citrate) during the remaining 76 days.

Zoledronic acid significantly reduces the risk of vertebral, hip, and other fractures. It is administered intravenously (5 mg) annually and has been evaluated in the treatment of postmenopausal osteoporosis.

Strontium ranelate

Like calcium, strontium is an alkaline earth element (group II in the periodic table), and is thus incorporated into the skeleton. Randomized, controlled trials have shown a decreased risk of vertebral and hip fractures with strontium ranelate. The dose is one 2 g sachet per day. It can cause diarrhoea, but this resolves on stopping treatment. There appears to be a small increased risk (less than 1%) of venous thromboembolism and nervous system disorders (headaches, seizures, memory loss and disturbance in consciousness), but further data are required. Like bisphosphonates, strontium ranelate is not advised in women with fertility aspirations, since the effects on the fetal skeleton are unknown.

Strontium ranelate causes a clinically significant overestimation of BMD because of the high attenuation of X-rays by strontium atoms in bone, as it has a higher atomic number (38) than calcium (20). Corrections are being studied to allow interpretation of BMD measurements in patients taking strontium ranelate.

Raloxifene

Raloxifene is a selective oestrogen receptor modulator (SERM). These compounds possess oestrogenic actions in certain tissues and anti-oestrogenic actions in others. Raloxifene is licensed for the prevention of osteoporosis-related vertebral fracture. It reduces vertebral but not non-vertebral fractures by 30–50%, depending on the dose. The standard dose is 60 mg/day. It also reduces the risk of breast cancer to the same extent as tamoxifen. Side-effects include hot flushes and calf cramps. It was thought that it could be cardioprotective from its effects on lipids; however, the Raloxifene Use for the Heart (RUTH) study found that it did not reduce the risk of coronary heart disease, and that it increased the risk of fatal stroke and venous thromboembolism. New SERMs, such as bazedoxifene, arzoxifene, lasofoxifene and ospemifene, are currently being evaluated.

Parathyroid hormone peptides

Recombinant 1–34 parathyroid hormone, given as a subcutaneous daily injection of 20 μg, reduces vertebral and non-vertebral fractures in post-menopausal women with osteoporosis. The full 1–84 parathyroid hormone peptide is given in the same way in a daily dose of 100 μg. They both reduce the risk of vertebral but not hip fractures. Because they cost more than other options, they are reserved for patients with severe osteoporosis who are unable to tolerate or seem to be unresponsive to other treatments.

Calcitonin

Calcitonin can be given by subcutaneous or intramuscular injection or by nasal spray. Nasal calcitonin has also been shown to reduce new vertebral fractures in women with established osteoporosis. Evidence exists for its efficacy as an analgesic in acute vertebral fracture. It may also be helpful as adjunctive treatment after surgery for hip fracture. An oral preparation is being developed.

Calcitriol

Calcitriol, the active metabolite of vitamin D, facilitates the intestinal absorption of calcium. It also has direct effects on bone cells. Studies of the effects of calcitriol on bone loss and fractures have produced conflicting results. The potential dangers of hypercalcaemia and hypercalciuria mean that levels of calcium in serum and urine should be monitored closely, so its use is limited.

Non-pharmacological interventions

Calcium and vitamin D

Provision of adequate dietary or supplemental calcium and vitamin D is an essential part of osteoporosis management (Table 9.2). In northern latitudes, cutaneous synthesis of vitamin D occurs only in the summer, and many diets lack sufficient amounts of this vitamin for adequate intake in the absence of solar exposure. Most studies show that about 1.5 g of elemental calcium is necessary to preserve bone health in postmenopausal women and elderly women who are not taking hormone replacement therapy. The effects of calcium and vitamin D supplements alone or in combination on fracture, however, are contradictory and may depend on the study population and compliance with therapy. For example, people in sheltered accommodation or residential care may be more frail, have lower dietary intakes of calcium and vitamin D, and are at higher risk of fracture than those living in the community.

Caution has been expressed about the use of supplements in women whose diet is replete (Table 9.2). The Women's Health Initiative study showed an increase in kidney stones and an RCT of 1471 women found upward trends in cardiovascular event rates in low-risk women taking calcium and vitamin D supplements.

Hip protectors

Hip protectors are used to reduce the impact of falling directly on the hip, but evidence of efficacy on fracture is conflicting in both the community and institutional settings. Systematic review has found no evidence of the effectiveness of hip protectors from studies in which randomization was by individual patient within an institution or for those living in their own homes.

Table 9.2

Calcium content of some foods

Food	Calcium content (mg)
Full-fat milk (250 ml)	295
Semi-skimmed milk (250 ml)	300
Skimmed milk (250 ml)	305
Low-fat yogurt (100 g)	150
Cheddar cheese (50 g)	360
Boiled spinach (100 g)	159
Brazil nuts (100 g)	170
Tinned salmon (100 g)	93
Tofu (100 g)	480

Future developments

New treatments are focusing on inhibition of bone turnover. Receptor activator of nuclear factor-κB ligand (RANKL) is a pivotal regulator of osteoclast activity that provides a new therapeutic target. Early studies have demonstrated that denosumab, an investigational, highly specific anti-RANKL antibody, rapidly and substantially reduces bone resorption. Pharmacokinetics of the antibody allow dosing by subcutaneous injection at an interval of 3 or 6 months. Data so far are encouraging.

Further reading

Bisphosphonates

Basu N, Reid DM. Bisphosphonate-associated osteonecrosis of the jaw. *Menopause Int* 2007;**13**:56–9.

Black DM, Delmas PD, Eastell R, *et al.*; HORIZON Pivotal Fracture Trial. Once-yearly zoledronic acid for treatment of postmenopausal osteoporosis. *N Engl J Med* 2007;**356**:1809–22.

Black DM, Schwartz AV, Ensrud KE, *et al.*; FLEX Research Group. Effects of continuing or stopping alendronate after 5 years of treatment: the Fracture Intervention Trial Long-Term Extension (FLEX): a randomized trial. *JAMA* 2006;**296**:2927–38.

Lyles KW, Colón-Emeric CS, Magaziner JS, *et al.*; HORIZON Recurrent Fracture Trial. Zoledronic acid and clinical fractures and mortality after hip fracture. *N Engl J Med* 2007;**357**:1799–1809.

Poole KES, Compston JE. Osteoporosis and its management. *BMJ* 2006;**333**:1251–6.

Recker RR, Kendler D, Recknor CP, *et al.* Comparative effects of raloxifene and alendronate on fracture outcomes in postmenopausal women with low bone mass. *Bone* 2007;**40**:843–51.

Silverman SL, Watts NB, Delmas PD, *et al.* Effectiveness of bisphosphonates on nonvertebral and hip fractures in the first year of therapy: the risedronate and alendronate (REAL) cohort study. *Osteoporos Int* 2007;**18**:25–34.

Sørensen HT, Christensen S, Mehnert F, *et al.* Use of bisphosphonates among women and risk of atrial fibrillation and flutter: population based case-control study. *BMJ* 2008;**336**:813–16.

Strontium ranelate and parathyroid hormone

Blake GM, Fogelman I. Effect of bone strontium on BMD measurements. *J Clin Densitom* 2007;**10**:34–8.

Greenspan SL, Bone HG, Ettinger MP, *et al.*; Treatment of Osteoporosis with Parathyroid Hormone Study Group. Effect of recombinant human parathyroid hormone (1–84) on vertebral fracture and bone mineral density in postmenopausal women with osteoporosis: a randomized trial. *Ann Intern Med* 2007;**146**:326–39.

Neer RM, Arnaud CD, Zanchetta JR, *et al.* Effect of parathyroid hormone on vertebral bone mass and fracture incidence among postmenopausal women with osteoporosis. *N Engl J Med* 2001;**344**:1434–41.

O'Donnell S, Cranney A, Wells GA, *et al.* Strontium ranelate for preventing and treating postmenopausal osteoporosis. *Cochrane Database Syst Rev* 2006;**3**:CD005326.

Roux C. Antifracture efficacy of strontium ranelate in postmenopausal osteoporosis. *Bone* 2007;**40**: S9–11.

Selective oestrogen receptor modulators

Barrett-Connor E, Mosca L, Collins P, *et al.*; Raloxifene Use for The Heart (RUTH) Trial Investigators. Effects of raloxifene on cardiovascular events and breast cancer in postmenopausal women. *N Engl J Med* 2006;**355**:125–37.

Palacios S. The future of the new selective estrogen receptor modulators. *Menopause Int* 2007;**13**:27–34.

Vogel VG, Costantino JP, Wickerham DL, *et al.*; National Surgical Adjuvant Breast and Bowel Project (NSABP). Effects of tamoxifen vs raloxifene on the risk of developing invasive breast cancer and other disease outcomes: the NSABP Study of Tamoxifen and Raloxifene (STAR) P-2 trial. *JAMA* 2006;**295**:2727–41.

Calcitonin and calcitriol

Chapuy MC, Arlot ME, Duboeuf F, *et al.* Vitamin D_3 and calcium to prevent hip fractures in elderly women. *N Engl J Med* 1992;**327**:1637–42.

Knopp JA, Diner BM, Blitz M, *et al.* Calcitonin for treating acute pain of osteoporotic vertebral compression fractures: a systematic review of randomized, controlled trials. *Osteoporos Int* 2005;**16**:1281–90.

Munoz-Torres M, Alonso G, Raya MP. Calcitonin therapy in osteoporosis. *Treat Endocrinol* 2004;**3**:117–32.

Tanko LB, Bagger YZ, Alexandersen P, *et al.* Safety and efficacy of a novel salmon calcitonin (sCT) technology-based oral formulation in healthy postmenopausal women: acute and 3-month effects on biomarkers of bone turnover. *J Bone Miner Res* 2004;**19**:1531–8.

Tilyard MW, Spears GFS, Thomson J, Dovey S. Treatment of postmenopausal osteoporosis with calcitriol or calcium. *N Engl J Med* 1992;**326**:357–62.

Calcium and vitamin D

Bischoff-Ferrari HA, Willett WC, Wong JB, *et al.* Fracture prevention with vitamin D supplementation: a meta-analysis of randomized controlled trials. *JAMA* 2005;**293**:2257–64.

Bolland MJ, Barber PA, Doughty RN, *et al.* Vascular events in healthy older women receiving calcium supplementation: randomised controlled trial. *BMJ* 2008;**336**: 262–6.

Grant AM, Avenell A, Campbell MK, *et al*. Oral vitamin D_3 and calcium for secondary prevention of low-trauma fractures in elderly people (Randomised Evaluation of Calcium or Vitamin D, RECORD): a randomised placebo-controlled trial. *Lancet* 2005;**365**:1621–8.

Jackson RD, LaCroix AZ, Gass M, *et al*.; Women's Health Initiative Investigators. Calcium plus vitamin D supplementation and the risk of fractures. *N Engl J Med* 2006;**354**:669–83.

Optimal Calcium Intake. National Institutes of Health. Consensus Development Conference Statement June 6–8, 1994. consensus.nih.gov/1994/1994Optimal Calcium097html.htm.

Porthouse J, Cockayne S, King C, *et al*. Randomised controlled trial of calcium and supplementation with cholecalciferol (vitamin D_3) for prevention of fractures in primary care. *BMJ* 2005;**330**:1003–6.

Prince RL. Calcium and vitamin D – for whom and when. *Menopause Int* 2007;**13**: 35–7.

Reginster JY. The high prevalence of inadequate serum vitamin D levels and implications for bone health. *Curr Med Res Opin* 2005;**21**:579–86.

Shea B, Wells G, Cranney A, *et al*. Calcium supplementation on bone loss in postmenopausal women. *Cochrane Database Syst Rev* 2004;**1**:CD004526.

Tang BM, Eslick GD, Nowson C, *et al*. Use of calcium or calcium in combination with vitamin D supplementation to prevent fractures and bone loss in people aged 50 years and older: a meta-analysis. *Lancet* 2007;**370**:657–66.

Hip protectors

Birks YF, Porthouse J, Addie C, *et al*.; Primary Care Hip Protector Trial Group. Randomized controlled trial of hip protectors among women living in the community. *Osteoporos Int* 2004;**15**:701–6.

Kiel DP, Magaziner J, Zimmerman S, *et al*. Efficacy of a hip protector to prevent hip fracture in nursing home residents: the HIP PRO randomized controlled trial. *JAMA* 2007;**298**:413–22.

Parker MJ, Gillespie WJ, Gillespie LD. Effectiveness of hip protectors for preventing hip fractures in elderly people: systematic review. *BMJ* 2006;**332**:571–4.

Future developments

Lewiecki EM, Miller PD, McClung MR, *et al*.; AMG 162 Bone Loss Study Group. Two-year treatment with denosumab (AMG 162) in a randomized phase 2 study of postmenopausal women with low BMD. *J Bone Miner Res* 2007;**22**:1832–41.

McClung M. Role of RANKL inhibition in osteoporosis. *Arthritis Res Ther* 2007;**9**(Suppl 1):S3.

10 Diet, lifestyle and exercise

Diet
Exercise
Smoking cessation
Further reading

Diet

The role of diet is of increasing interest and not only in the prevention of obesity. Older people are more vulnerable to inadequate nutrition, which leads to the anorexia of ageing and gradual weight loss. Poor nutritional status is associated with increased demands on health services, lengthier hospital stays and immune dysfunction, and it is recognized as an important predictor of morbidity and mortality.

Moreover, different diets appear to have health benefits. Studies consistently support the view that the Mediterranean diet is compatible with healthier ageing and increased longevity. It may also lower the risk of obesity, metabolic syndrome, type 2 diabetes and dementia. The Mediterranean diet is characterized by high intake of vegetables, legumes, fruits and cereals (in the past largely unrefined); moderate to high intake of fish; low intake of saturated lipids but high intake of unsaturated lipids, particularly olive oil; low to moderate intake of dairy products, mostly cheese and yogurt; low intake of meat; and modest intake of alcohol, mostly as wine. Mediterranean and modified Mediterranean diets are associated with reductions in mortality. The benefit of the diet does not seem to be limited to Mediterranean countries and can be exported to others.

The American Heart Association recommends that 'Women should consume a diet rich in fruits and vegetables; choose whole-grain, high-fiber foods; consume fish, especially oily fish, at least twice a week; limit intake of saturated fat to <10% of energy, and if possible to <7%, cholesterol to <300 mg/d, alcohol intake to no more than 1 drink per day, and sodium intake to <2.3 g/d (approximately 1 tsp salt). Consumption of *trans*-fatty acids should be as low as possible (eg <1% of energy)'.

Dietary components

Macronutrients

Macronutrients encompass carbohydrates, protein and fat. While there are dietary recommendations for older people, it is important that the diet be compatible with alterations in perceptions of taste and dentition with age and concomitant diseases, such as diabetes, and drug therapy, such as warfarin.

Carbohydrates

The World Health Organization (WHO) recommends that 55–75% of energy input come from carbohydrates, with less than 10% from free sugars. As diets high in non-milk extrinsic sugars may reduce intake of foods that are more nutrient dense, these should be eaten in moderation. More emphasis is needed on other carbohydrate-rich foods (such as whole-grain breakfast cereal, bread and other bakery products), which would also provide fibre and a number of B vitamins. Furthermore, diets high in whole grains are associated with lower BMI and smaller waist measurement as well as lower risk of developing metabolic syndrome.

Protein

Protein is an important nutrient for the older woman. Current recommendations are 10–15% of total energy intake. As lean body mass decreases with age, it would seem intuitively that protein requirements would decline, but instead they increase to maintain nitrogen equilibrium. Demand further increases in wound healing (including fractures), infection and restoring muscle mass lost from immobility.

Fat

The WHO recommends that total fat intake should account for 15–30% of total energy intake, with saturated fats accounting for less than 10% and polyunsaturated fats for 6–10%. Although the main message in the past has been to limit the total amount of fat, particular types, such as omega-3 fatty acids, which are found mainly in oily fish, may be more important than previously recognized (see below). The Women's Health Initiative randomized, controlled trial examined the effect of reduction of total fat intake on the risk of breast and colorectal cancer and cardiovascular disease (CVD). In this study, 16,541 women were assigned to a diet with reduced total fat intake (20% total energy) and increased intakes of vegetables, fruit and grains. The comparison group of 29,294 women did not have any dietary changes. Mean follow-up was 8.1 years. The dietary intervention had no effect.

Micronutrients

Micronutrients encompass vitamins and minerals. The role of calcium and vitamin D is discussed in Chapter 9. The significant micronutrients that may be associated with deficiencies in elderly women include vitamin B_{12}, vitamin A, vitamin C, vitamin D, zinc and other trace minerals. Low intake of a range of micronutrients, such as iron, folate and vitamin B_{12}, can cause a number of anaemias and a range of other problems (such as neuropathies and dementia).

It has been suggested that antioxidant supplements may reduce mortality. However, systematic review has found that vitamin A, beta-carotene, and vitamin E supplements may increase mortality. No detrimental effects were found with vitamin C or selenium. Of note, most trials in the systematic review investigated the effects of supplements administered at higher doses than those commonly found in a balanced diet, and some of the trials used doses above the recommended daily allowances. These trials should not deter women from consuming fruit and vegetables, which contain other substances such as fibre and flavonoids. Increased intake of vegetables, as in the Mediterranean diet, appears to be associated with reduced mortality.

Vitamin A

Vitamin A has many roles in the maintenance of health. It is important for normal vision, cell differentiation, immune function and genetic expression. Higher serum levels of carotenoids are associated with a lower mortality in older women. However, high vitamin A intake is associated with higher risk of fracture, as it is a vitamin D and calcium antagonist. Consuming a diet rich in fruit and vegetables is a reasonable way to meet vitamin A needs, and these foods are a good source of dietary fibre.

Vitamin B_{12} (cobalamin) and folate

Vitamin B_{12} (cobalamin) deficiency can lead to macrocytic anaemias and neuropathies. Dietary sources of vitamin B_{12} are primarily meats and dairy products. Folates are found in fruit and fresh vegetables. Deficiency may also lead to macrocytic anaemia and neurological problems. It is important to distinguish between cobalamin and folate deficiency, since supplementation with folate may delay the diagnosis and worsen the sequelae of cobalamin deficiency. Cobalamin and folate are involved in homocysteine metabolism. High homocysteine levels have been suggested as risk factors for cognitive decline, dementia, CVD and osteoporotic fracture. However, a randomized, controlled trial of a combination pill of folic acid, vitamin B_6, and vitamin B_{12} has not reduced a combined endpoint of total cardiovascular events among high-risk women, despite significant homocysteine lowering. Gender differences may exist, in that lower bone mineral density (BMD) has been associated with higher homocysteine levels in women, but not in men.

Vitamin C

Low blood concentrations of vitamin C in men and women aged 75–84 years are predictive of mortality. Vitamin C status is generally related to dietary intake, the main source being fruit and vegetables. However, high intake of vitamin C from supplements is associated with increased risk of mortality from CVD in postmenopausal women with diabetes.

Vitamin E

Although one study showed that vitamin E reduced hot flushes, the difference between the active and placebo groups was not significant. Vitamin E does not reduce the risk of CVD or cancer, and supplement use is associated with increased mortality.

Vitamin K

It is now apparent that vitamin K not only affects blood clotting but also plays a role in bone metabolism and potential protection against osteoporosis. Vitamin K is required for the gamma-carboxylation of osteocalcin. Epidemiological studies and clinical trials indicate that vitamin K has a positive effect on BMD and decreases fracture risk. Typical dietary intakes of vitamin K are below the levels associated with better BMD and reduced fracture risk; thus, issues of increasing dietary intake, supplementation, and/or fortification arise. Large-scale, intervention trials of vitamin K are needed to address these issues. This has implications for the use of coumarin-based anticoagulants such as warfarin, and studies suggest that long-term therapy adversely affects vertebral BMD and fracture risk. Vegetables, particularly dark green, leafy vegetables, are the most important source of vitamin K.

Trace elements
Selenium

Selenium is an essential nutrient that enhances immune function and increases antioxidant activity. Its level in food reflects the soil in which it was grown and therefore varies worldwide. Low levels of selenium are associated with increased risk of mortality. There is an upper limit of about 450 μg of selenium per day, which, if exceeded, may lead to toxicity. Symptoms of toxicity include nausea, vomiting, hair and nail brittleness and loss, irritability, peripheral neuropathy, and fatigue.

Magnesium

Hypomagnesaemia has been considered as a possible factor in depressed immune function, muscle atrophy, osteoporosis, hyperglycaemia, hyperlipidaemia, and other neuromuscular, cardiovascular, or renal dysfunctions. The role of magnesium in dementia has been a recent focus of attention. Food sources include green, leafy, vegetables, unpolished grains, nuts, meat, starches and milk.

Zinc

Zinc is another essential trace nutrient: it is essential for neurogenesis and plays an important role in neurotransmission. Consequences of poor zinc status may include reduced immune function, dermatitis, loss of taste acuity, impaired wound healing, and impaired cognitive function. Food sources include fortified cereals, red meat and certain seafoods.

Functional foods

A functional food may be defined as a food having health-promoting benefits and/or disease-preventing properties over and above its usual nutritional value. Functional foods are also known as 'nutraceuticals' or 'designer foods'. Functional foods encompass a broad range of products, ranging from foods generated around a particular functional ingredient (eg stanol-enriched margarine), through to staples fortified with a nutrient that would not normally be present to any great extent (eg folic acid-fortified bread or breakfast cereal). Functional foods were developed and first regulated in Japan in the 1980s, and then spread to northern Europe and North America. Regulations regarding statements about the beneficial effect of a food or its ingredients on health vary throughout the world. In Europe, claims that a food can treat, prevent or cure a disease (medical claims) are still prohibited.

There are concerns about interaction of functional foods with standard drugs, and about consumption affecting compliance. Functional foods cannot be considered to replace medication, and advice from a health professional should be sought. For example, phytosterols and stanols interact with statins and have an additive effect on reducing low-density lipoprotein cholesterol (LDL-C) values. However, while statins and phytosterols, and stanols can be taken together, a lower dose of statins cannot be compensated for by the intake of functional foods.

Functional foods that show promise in women's health include the following:

- probiotics
- prebiotics
- phytosterols and stanols
- omega-3 fatty acids
- flavonoids
- fibre.

Isoflavones can also be considered as a functional food, as discussed in Chapter 11. Synbiotics are a food or supplement product containing both probiotics and prebiotics. The name derives from a proposed synergism between probiotics and prebiotics.

Probiotics

Probiotics are live micro-organisms that, when administered in adequate amounts, confer a health benefit on the host. The concept of probiotics emerged from observations in the 19th century by the Russian immunologist Elie Metchnikoff, who hypothesized that the long, healthy lives of Bulgarian peasants were rooted in their consumption of fermented milk containing beneficial *Lactobacillus*, and the positive influence of these microbes on colonic health. It is now apparent that micro-organisms have an important influence on immune development and resistance to infection. Currently, the best-studied probiotics are different species of *Lactobacillus* or *Bifidobacterium*, and the yeast *Saccharomyces cerevisiae* (boulardii). These can be combined in cereals, bars, yohurt and drinks. Various health benefits have been proposed, such as regulation of immune function, improvement of inflammatory bowel conditions, shortening the duration of infectious diarrhoea in infants, enhanced gastrointestinal tolerance of antibiotic therapy, and control of symptoms associated with lactose intolerance. They may also improve therapeutic outcome for women being treated for bacterial vaginosis and reduce the severity of the symptoms or the incidence of respiratory infections.

Prebiotics

Prebiotics are indigestible food ingredients that beneficially affect the host by selectively stimulating the growth and/or activity of one or a limited number of bacteria in the colon. Thus, prebiotics are food for bacterial species that are considered beneficial for health and wellbeing. The bacterial species primarily of interest include those in the *Lactobacillus* and *Bifidobacterium* genera. This criterion is currently fulfilled only by some indigestible but fermentable carbohydrates (inulin and certain oligosaccharides).

Phytosterols and stanols

Phytosterols and stanols reduce LDL-C by 10% and thus have the potential of reducing the risk of coronary heart disease (CHD) by about 25%. However, studies with the endpoints of cardiovascular events are awaited. Plant sterols and stanols reduce the absorption of cholesterol from the gut and so lower serum concentrations of cholesterol. Dietary sources include vegetable oils, nuts, seeds and grains, but the amounts are often not large enough to have significant cholesterol-lowering effects. Dietary intake does not usually exceed 250–300 mg/day in northern European countries, whereas it appears to be higher (up to 500–600 mg/day) in Mediterranean countries. These agents have been extracted from tall (derived from the process of paper production from wood) and/or soy oil and were traditionally incorporated in foods with higher fat content, such as spreads and salad dressings. More recently, they have also been incorporated in low-fat foods, including bread and cereal, low-fat milk, and low-fat yogurt.

Omega-3 fatty acids

Omega-3 fatty acids include the plant-derived alpha-linolenic acid (ALA, 18:3n-3), and the fish-oil-derived eicosapentaenoic acid (EPA, 20:5n-3) and docoshexaenoic acid (DHA, 22:6n-3). Observational studies such as the Nurses' Health Study have shown a reduction in CVD in consumers of oily fish. The cardioprotective effects of omega-3 fatty acids are thought to result partly from the hypotriglycerolaemic effects of EPA and DHA. Consumption of a diet rich in omega-3 fatty acids may also protect against dementia and Alzheimer's disease.

Flavonoids

Flavonoids are a large family of polyphenolic compounds synthesized by plants. They are found in a wide variety of fruit and vegetables such as grapes, berries, apples, chocolate, tea, kale and hot peppers. Isoflavones are a subclass of flavonoids with oestrogenic activity, as discussed in Chapter 11. Epidemiological evidence suggests that flavonoids reduce the risk of CVD. This would explain the inverse relationship between the consumption of red wine and CVD mortality (the French paradox). Possible mechanisms include a reduction in platelet activation, inflammation and LDL oxidation, and improvement of endothelial function. Animal and *in vitro* studies suggest that flavonoids may have a role in preventing cancer and neurodegenerative disease.

Fibre

Dietary fibre consists of plant substances that resist hydrolysis by digestive enzymes in the small bowel; it is an extremely complex group of substances. Fibre can be classified according to its solubility and fermentability by bacteria: soluble fibre is readily fermentable by colonic bacteria, while insoluble fibre is only slowly fermentable. Fibres may act in several ways, including through gel-forming effects in the stomach and small intestine, fermentation by colonic bacteria, a 'mop and sponge' effect, and concomitant changes in other aspects of the diet. These actions lead to potentially beneficial effects in the gastrointestinal tract and systemically, such as lowering levels of cholesterol in serum and improving glycaemic control. Dietary fibre intake may modulate parameters associated with the control of the metabolic syndrome, namely food intake (and body weight), glycaemia and insulinaemia, blood lipids and blood pressure.

Maintaining optimal weight and BMI

One of the outcomes noted in the Nurses' Health Study was that there is a gradient of coronary risk, with the heaviest category of women having a threefold risk of CHD compared with lean women. Much evidence has focused on the distribution of fat, with a more android morphology (apple) representing a higher cardiac risk than a more gynoid (pear) shape. Thus, a waist circumference of 76.2 cm (30 in) or more was associated with more than a twofold higher risk of CHD. The American Heart Association recommends that 'Women should maintain or lose weight through an appropriate balance of physical activity, caloric intake, and formal behavioral programs when indicated to maintain/achieve a BMI between 18.5 and 24.9 kg/m^2 and a waist circumference ≤35 in'. In the UK, the National Health Service has similar recommendations. However, recommendations may vary between different ethnic groups. Pharmacological therapy should be considered as an adjunct to diet and lifestyle changes. Current licensed anti-obesity drugs include orlistat, sibutramine and rimonobant.

Exercise

Regular physical activity reduces the risk of CHD, osteoporotic fractures and type 2 diabetes mellitus. Hot flushes, urinary incontinence, insomnia and depression may also be helped. A systematic review found that no conclusions regarding the effectiveness of exercise as a treatment for vasomotor menopausal symptoms could be made due to a lack of trials.

Exercise and coronary heart disease

Lower fitness levels are associated with a 4.7-fold increased risk of CHD. The reported beneficial effect of exercise on CHD risk profile are less marked in women than men, with smaller increases in high-density lipoprotein cholesterol and less weight loss resulting from similar exercise training. However, the Nurses' Health Study found that low-intensity exercise, such as walking, conferred the same benefit as vigorous exercise, and sedentary women who became active late in life reaped similar benefits as those who remained active throughout.

Exercise, falls prevention and osteoporotic fracture

Exercise has a key role in the prevention and treatment of osteoporosis. Exercise can provide overall increases in strength, flexibility and balance, with diminished risk of falling. Exercise increases BMD. Various types of exercise are used; however, what types, intensity, frequency and duration of activity are most effective is unclear. They include weight bearing, back extension, Tai Chi, Pilates and vibration exercise. Physical activity not only is an important determinant of peak bone mass but also helps to maintain bone mass in later life. A Cochrane Review found that fast walking effectively improved bone density in the spine and the hip, whereas weight-bearing exercises were associated with increases in bone density of the spine, but not the hip. Exercise regimens can be very helpful in the management of established osteoporosis and are a component of falls prevention programmes.

Pelvic floor exercises

Pelvic floor exercises are used commonly for stress incontinence. They are also used in the treatment of women with mixed incontinence, and less commonly for urge incontinence. Adjuncts, such as biofeedback or electrical stimulation, are also commonly used with training of the muscle of the pelvic floor. Studies have different designs and endpoints of treatment (self-reported or objective assessment). Systematic reviews support the view that pelvic floor muscle training and bladder training should be included in first-line conservative management programmes for women with stress, urge, or mixed, urinary incontinence.

Smoking cessation

Smoking increases mortality in women from CVD, pulmonary disease, lung cancer, and other cancers such as colorectal cancer. The Nurses' Health Study found that that 64% of deaths in current smokers and 28% of deaths in past smokers are attributable to smoking. Stopping smoking reduced the excess mortality rates for all major causes of death examined. Most of the excess risk of vascular mortality due to smoking may be eliminated rapidly upon cessation and within 20 years for lung disease. Early age at initiation of smoking is associated with increased mortality.

With regard to CHD, compared to non-smokers, female current smokers have a relative risk of myocardial infarction of 2.24 (range 1.85–2.71). Second-hand smoke also increases the risk of CHD.

The INTERHEART case-control study estimated that 29% of heart attack cases in Western Europe are due to smoking, and smokers and former smokers are at almost twice the risk of a heart attack as never smokers.

Further reading

General references

British Nutrition Foundation. www.nutrition.org.uk.

Buckland G, Bach A, Serra-Majem L. Obesity and the Mediterranean diet: a systematic review of observational and intervention studies. *Obes Rev* 2008;**9**:582–93.

Fabian E, Elmadfa I. Nutritional situation of the elderly in the European Union: data of the European Nutrition and Health Report (2004). *Ann Nutr Metab* 2008;**52**(Suppl 1):57–61.

Food and Nutrition Information Center, National Agricultural Library, United States Department of Agriculture. Dietary Guidance. fnic.nal.usda.gov/nal.

Giugliano D, Esposito K. Mediterranean diet and metabolic diseases. *Curr Opin Lipidol* 2008;**19**:63–8.

Knoops KT, de Groot LC, Kromhout D, *et al.* Mediterranean diet, lifestyle factors, and 10-year mortality in elderly European men and women: the HALE project. *JAMA* 2004;**292**:1433–9.

Martínez-González MA, de la Fuente-Arrillaga C, Nunez-Cordoba JM, *et al.* Adherence to Mediterranean diet and risk of developing diabetes: prospective cohort study. *BMJ* 2008;**336**:1348–51.

Mosca L, Banka CL, Benjamin EJ, *et al.* Evidence-based guidelines for cardiovascular disease prevention in women: 2007 update. *Circulation* 2007;**115**:1481–501.

Salerno-Kennedy R, Cashman KD. The role of nutrition in dementia: an overview. *J Br Menopause Soc* 2006;**12**:44–8.

Trichopoulou A, Orfanos P, Norat T, *et al.* Modified Mediterranean diet and survival: EPIC-elderly prospective cohort study. *BMJ* 2005;**330**:991.

World Health Organization. Diet, nutrition and the prevention of chronic diseases. Report of the joint WHO/FAO expert consultation. 2003 WHO Technical Report Series, no. 916 (TRS 916). www.who.int/dietphysicalactivity/publications/trs916/en.

Macronutrients

Beresford SA, Johnson KC, Ritenbaugh C, *et al.* Low-fat dietary pattern and risk of colorectal cancer: the Women's Health Initiative Randomized Controlled Dietary Modification Trial. *JAMA* 2006;**295**:643–54.

Good CK, Holschuh N, Albertson AM, Eldridge AL. Whole grain consumption and body mass index in adult women: an analysis of NHANES 1999–2000 and the USDA pyramid servings database. *J Am Coll Nutr* 2008;**27**:80–7.

Heaney RP, Layman DK. Amount and type of protein influences bone health. *Am J Clin Nutr* 2008;**87**:1567S–70S.

Howard BV, Van Horn L, Hsia J, *et al.* Low-fat dietary pattern and risk of cardiovascular disease: the Women's Health Initiative Randomized Controlled Dietary Modification Trial. *JAMA* 2006;**295**:655–66.

Prentice RL, Caan B, Chlebowski RT, *et al.* Low-fat dietary pattern and risk of invasive breast cancer: the Women's Health Initiative Randomized Controlled Dietary Modification Trial. *JAMA* 2006;**295**:629–42.

Sahyoun NR, Jacques PF, Zhang XL, *et al.* Whole-grain intake is inversely associated with the metabolic syndrome and mortality in older adults. *Am J Clin Nutr* 2006;**83**:124–31.

Micronutrients

Agudo A, Cabrera L, Amiano P, *et al.* Fruit and vegetable intakes, dietary antioxidant nutrients, and total mortality in Spanish adults: findings from the Spanish cohort of the European Prospective Investigation into Cancer and Nutrition (EPIC-Spain). *Am J Clin Nutr* 2007;**85**:1634–42.

Albert CM, Cook NR, Gaziano JM, *et al.* Effect of folic acid and B vitamins on risk of cardiovascular events and total mortality among women at high risk for cardiovascular disease: a randomized trial. *JAMA* 2008;**299**:2027–36.

Balducci L, Ershler WB, Krantz S. Anemia in the elderly – clinical findings and impact on health. *Crit Rev Oncol Hematol* 2006;**58**:156–65.

Barton DL, Loprinzi CL, Quella SK, *et al.* Prospective evaluation of vitamin E for hot flashes in breast cancer survivors. *J Clin Oncol* 1998;**16**:495–500.

Bhatnagar S, Taneja S. Zinc and cognitive development. *Br J Nutr* 2001;**85**(Suppl 2):S139–45.

Bjelakovic G, Nikolova D, Gluud L, *et al.* Antioxidant supplements for prevention of mortality in healthy participants and patients with various diseases. *Cochrane Database Syst Rev* 2008;**2**:CD007176.

Chernoff R. Micronutrient requirements in older women. *Am J Clin Nutr* 2005;**81**: 1240S–5S.

Cilliler AE, Ozturk S, Ozbakir S. Serum magnesium level and clinical deterioration in Alzheimer's disease. *Gerontology* 2007;**53**:419–22.

Fletcher AE, Breeze E, Shetty PS. Antioxidant vitamins and mortality in older persons: findings from the nutrition add-on study to the Medical Research Council Trial of Assessment and Management of Older People in the Community. *Am J Clin Nutr* 2003;**78**:999–1010.

Gjesdal CG, Vollset SE, Ueland PM, *et al.* Plasma total homocysteine level and bone mineral density: the Hordaland Homocysteine Study. *Arch Intern Med* 2006;**166**: 88–94.

Lauretani F, Semba RD, Bandinelli S, *et al.* Low plasma selenium concentrations and mortality among older community-dwelling adults: the InCHIANTI Study. *Aging Clin Exp Res* 2008;**20**:153–8.

Lee IM, Cook NR, Gaziano JM, *et al.* Vitamin E in the primary prevention of cardiovascular disease and cancer: the Women's Health Study: a randomized controlled trial. *JAMA* 2005;**294**:56–65.

Lee DH, Folsom AR, Harnack L, *et al.* Does supplemental vitamin C increase cardiovascular disease risk in women with diabetes? *Am J Clin Nutr* 2004;**80**: 1194–1200.

Lonn E, Bosch J, Yusuf S, *et al.* Effects of long-term vitamin E supplementation on cardiovascular events and cancer: a randomized controlled trial. *JAMA* 2005;**293**:1338–47.

Miller ER 3rd, Pastor-Barriuso R, Dalal D, *et al.* Meta-analysis: high-dosage vitamin E supplementation may increase all-cause mortality. *Ann Intern Med* 2005;**142**: 37–46.

Pearson DA. Bone health and osteoporosis: the role of vitamin K and potential antagonism by anticoagulants. *Nutr Clin Pract* 2007;**22**:517–44.

Ray AL, Semba RD, Walston J, *et al.* Low serum selenium and total carotenoids predict mortality among older women living in the community: the women's health and aging studies. *J Nutr* 2006;**136**:172–6.

Selhub J. The many facets of hyperhomocysteinemia: studies from the Framingham cohorts. *J Nutr* 2006;**136**:1726S–30S.

Vaquero MP. Magnesium and trace elements in the elderly: intake, status and recommendations. *J Nutr Health Aging* 2002;**6**:147–53.

White SC, Atchison KA, Gornbein JA, *et al.* Risk factors for fractures in older men and women: the Leisure World Cohort Study. *Gend Med* 2006;**3**:110–23.

Functional foods

Barberger-Gateau P, Raffaitin C, Letenneur L, *et al.* Dietary patterns and risk of dementia: the Three-City cohort study. *Neurology* 2007;**69**:1921–30.

Commission of the European Communities. Regulation (EC) No. 1924/2006 of the European Parliament and of the Council of 20 December 2006. Official Journal of the European Union L 404 of 30 December 2006. Brussels: Commission of the European Communities, 2006.

de Jong N, Klungel OH, Verhagen H, *et al.* Functional foods: the case for closer evaluation. *BMJ* 2007;**334**:1037–9.

de Vrese M, Marteau PR. Probiotics and prebiotics: effects on diarrhea. *J Nutr* 2007;**137**(Suppl 2):803S–11S.

de Vrese M, Schrezenmeir J. Probiotics, prebiotics, and synbiotics. *Adv Biochem Eng Biotechnol* 2008;**111**:1–66.

Douglas LC, Sanders ME. Probiotics and prebiotics in dietetics practice. *J Am Diet Assoc* 2008;**108**:510–21.

Erlund I, Koli R, Alfthan G, *et al.* Favorable effects of berry consumption on platelet function, blood pressure, and HDL cholesterol. *Am J Clin Nutr* 2008;**87**:323–31.

Hu FB, Bronner L, Willett WC, *et al.* Fish and omega-3 fatty acid intake and risk of coronary heart disease in women. *JAMA* 2002;**287**:1815–21.

Huntley AL. Grape flavonoids and menopausal health. *Menopause Int* 2007;**13**:165–9.

James SL, Muir JG, Curtis SL, Gibson PR. Dietary fibre: a roughage guide. *Intern Med J* 2003;**33**:291–6.

Järvinen R, Knekt P, Rissanen H, Reunanen A. Intake of fish and long-chain n-3 fatty acids and the risk of coronary heart mortality in men and women. *Br J Nutr* 2006;**95**:824–9.

Lang T. Functional foods. *BMJ* 2007;**334**:1015–16.

Law M. Plant sterol and stanol margarines and health. *BMJ* 2000;**320**:861–4.

Martikainen JA, Ottelin AM, Kiviniemi V, Gylling H. Plant stanol esters are potentially cost-effective in the prevention of coronary heart disease in men: Bayesian modelling approach. *Eur J Cardiovasc Prev Rehabil* 2007;**14**:265–72.

Rudkovska I. Functional foods for cardiovascular disease in women. *Menopause Int* 2008;**14**:63–9.

Weaver CM, Barnes S, Wyss JM, *et al*. Botanicals for age-related diseases: from field to practice. *Am J Clin Nutr* 2008;**87**:493S–7S.

Maintaining optimal weight and BMI

Manson JE, Willet WC, Stampfer MJ, *et al*. Body weight and mortality among women. *N Engl J Med* 1995;**333**:677–85.

National Institute of Health and Clinical Excellence. Obesity: the prevention, identification, assessment and management of overweight and obesity in adults and children. December 2006. www.nice.org.uk/guidance/CG43/guidance.

Rexrode KM, Carey VJ, Hennekens CH, *et al*. Abdominal adiposity and coronary heart disease in women. *JAMA* 1998;**280**:1843–8.

Yarnell JW, Patterson CC, Thomas HF, *et al*. Central obesity: predictive value of skinfold measurements for subsequent ischaemic heart disease at 14 years follow-up in the Caerphilly Study. *Int J Obes Relat Metab Disord* 2001;**25**:1546–9.

Exercise

Asikainen TM, Kukkonen-Harjula K, Miilunpalo S. Exercise for health for early postmenopausal women: a systematic review of randomised controlled trials. *Sports Med* 2004;**34**:753–78.

Blair SN, Kohl HW, Paffenbarger RS, *et al*. Physical fitness and all cause mortality: a prospective study of healthy men and women. *JAMA* 1989;**262**:2395–401.

Bonaiuti D, Shea B, Iovine R, *et al*. Exercise for preventing and treating osteoporosis in postmenopausal women. *Cochrane Database Syst Rev* 2003;**4**:CD0000333.

Bush TL, Fried LP, Barrett-Connor E. Cholesterol, lipoproteins and coronary heart disease in women. *Clin Chem* 1988;**34**:B60–70.

Cardinale M, Rittweger J. Vibration exercise makes your muscles and bones stronger: fact or fiction? *Menopause Int* 2006;**12**:12–18.

Daley A, MacArthur C, Mutrie N, Stokes-Lampard H. Exercise for vasomotor menopausal symptoms. *Cochrane Database Syst Rev* 2007;**4**:CD006108.

Hay-Smith EJ, Dumoulin C. Pelvic floor muscle training versus no treatment, or inactive control treatments, for urinary incontinence in women. *Cochrane Database Syst Rev* 2006;**1**:CD005654.

Laybourne AH, Biggs S, Martin FC. Falls exercise interventions and reduced falls rate: always in the patient's interest? *Age Ageing* 2008;**37**:10–13.

Lin JT, Lane JM. Nonpharmacologic management of osteoporosis to minimize fracture risk. *Nat Clin Pract Rheumatol* 2008;**4**:20–5.

Lindh-Astrand L, Nedstrand E, Wyon Y, Hammar M. Vasomotor symptoms and quality of life in previously sedentary postmenopausal women randomised to physical activity or estrogen therapy. *Maturitas* 2004;**48**:97–105.

Manson JE, Greenland P, LaCroix AZ, *et al*. Walking compared with vigorous exercise for the prevention of cardiovascular events in women. *N Engl J Med* 2002;**347**: 716–25.

Shamliyan TA, Kane RL, Wyman J, Wilt TJ. Systematic review: randomized, controlled trials of nonsurgical treatments for urinary incontinence in women. *Ann Intern Med* 2008;**148**:459–73.

Wayne PM, Kiel DP, Krebs DE, *et al*. The effects of Tai Chi on bone mineral density in postmenopausal women: a systematic review. *Arch Phys Med Rehabil* 2007;**88**: 673–80.

Smoking cessation

Allender S, Peto V, Scarborough P, *et al*. Coronary heart disease statistics 2007. London: British Heath Foundation. www.heartstats.org.

Kenfield SA, Stampfer MJ, Rosner BA, Colditz GA. Smoking and smoking cessation in relation to mortality in women. *JAMA* 2008;**299**:2037–47.

Prescott E, Hippe M, Schnohr P, *et al*. Smoking and risk of myocardial infarction in women and men: longitudinal population study. *BMJ* 1998;**316**:1043–7.

Yusaf S, Hawken S, Ounpuu S, *et al*. on behalf of the INTERHEART Study Investigators. Effect of potentially modifiable risk factors associated with myocardial infarction in 52 countries (the INTERHEART Study): case control study. *Lancet* 2004;**364**:937–52.

11 Complementary and alternative medicine

Botanicals
Homeopathy
Dehydroepiandrosterone
Progesterone transdermal creams
'Mechanical' therapies
Further reading

Evidence from randomized trials that complementary and alternative medicine (CAM) improves menopausal symptoms or has the same benefits as hormone replacement therapy (HRT) is poor. Very little well-designed research has been done. Studies may have limitations such as design, sample size and duration. However, many women use CAM in the belief that they are safer and 'more natural', especially with the concerns about the safety of oestrogen-based HRT after publication of the Women's Health Initiative study and the Million Women Study. In the UK, one in 10 adults has received CAM therapy from a practitioner in the past year. In the USA and Australia, more than half the women use some type of CAM during midlife.

Botanicals

A variety of botanicals are used by women. The evidence from clinical trials of beneficial effect on menopausal symptoms is limited and conflicting. Studies may use different products that are not chemically consistent, making comparison difficult. Moreover, the stability of individual chemicals may vary and can depend on the type of packaging. Herbs may contain many chemical compounds whose individual and combined effects are unknown (Box 11.1).

A major concern is use without consulting a health professional, leading to interaction with standard pharmacopoeia with potentially fatal consequences. Botanical and other dietary supplements can also interact with each other. Severe adverse reactions, including renal and liver failure and cancer, have been reported. Concern exists about the quality control of production. Some have been found to be contaminated, contain unlabelled ingredients

---

Box 11.1

Herbs used by menopausal women

Actaea racemosa (black cohosh)
Piper methysticum (kava kava)
Oenothera biennis (evening primrose)
Angelica sinensis (dong quai)
Ginkgo biloba (gingko)
Panax ginseng (ginseng)

Others, such as wild yam cream, St John's wort (*Hypericum perforatum*), *Agnus castus* (chasteberry), liquorice root, hops, milk thistle, Chinese herbal medicines, pollen extracts and valerian root

---

such as conventional medicines (steroids) or banned substances, or have different amounts of ingredients from those listed on the label. Moreover, some preparations contain high levels of heavy metals, such as arsenic, lead and mercury. While a European Union (EU) Directive on traditional herbal medicinal products was implemented in October 2005 in the UK, this will not cover preparations bought by women outside Europe.

Phytoestrogens: soy and red clover

Phytoestrogens are plant substances that have effects similar to those of oestrogens. Preparations vary from enriched foods, such as bread or drinks (soy milk), to more concentrated tablets. The most important groups are called isoflavones and lignans. The major isoflavones are genistein and daidzein. The major lignans are enterolactone and enterodiol.

Isoflavones are found in soybeans, chickpeas, red clover and probably other legumes (beans and peas). Oilseeds such as flaxseed are rich in lignans, and they also are found in cereal bran, whole cereals, vegetables, legumes and fruit.

The role of phytoestrogens has stimulated considerable interest, as people from populations that consume a diet high in isoflavones, such as the Japanese, seem to have lower rates of menopausal vasomotor symptoms; cardiovascular disease; osteoporosis; and breast, colon, endometrial and ovarian cancers. PHYTOS, ISOHEART and PHYTOPREVENT are EU studies examining the role of phytoestrogens in osteoporosis, heart disease and cancer. The American Heart Association does not recommend use of isoflavone supplements in food or pills to reduce the risk of cardiovascular disease. In contrast, soy products such as tofu, soy butter, soy nuts or some soy burgers should be beneficial to cardiovascular and overall health because of their high content of polyunsaturated fats, fibre, vitamins and minerals and low content of saturated fat.

With regard to menopausal symptoms, the evidence from randomized, placebo-controlled trials in Western populations is conflicting for soy and derivatives of red clover. Similarly, debate also surrounds the effects on lipoproteins, endothelial function, blood pressure, cognition and the endometrium. Endometrial hyperplasia has been reported in soy users. The isoflavone daidzein is metabolized extensively in the gut to the more oestrogenic secondary metabolite equol by the human gut microflora. That only 30% of Western populations excrete high levels of equol might account for the conflicting evidence provided by clinical trials.

Further well-designed, randomized trials are needed to determine the role and safety of phytoestrogen supplements in perimenopausal and post-menopausal women and those who have survived cancer.

Actaea racemosa (black cohosh)

Actaea racemosa (formerly known as *Cimicifuga racemosa*), a herbaceous perennial plant native to North America, is used widely to alleviate menopausal symptoms. Its use for menopausal problems is recognized by the WHO and German health authorities.

There is no consensus as to the mechanism by which it relieves hot flushes. Whether or not it has oestrogenic action is debated, with most data derived from *in vitro* or animal models, which cannot necessarily be extrapolated to man.

The results from placebo-controlled trials or comparison are conflicting, but little is known about the long-term safety, and liver toxicity has been reported.

Oenothera biennis (evening primrose)

Evening primrose oil is rich in gamma-linolenic acid. One small, placebo-controlled, randomized trial showed it to be ineffective for treating hot flushes.

Angelica sinensis (dong quai)

Dong quai is a perennial plant native to south-west China that is used commonly in traditional Chinese medicine. It was not found to be superior to placebo in a randomized trial but may be effective when combined with other herbs. Interaction with warfarin and photosensitization have been reported.

Ginkgo biloba (gingko)

The use of *Gingko biloba* is widespread, but there is little evidence that it improves menopausal symptoms.

Panax ginseng (ginseng)

Ginseng is a perennial herb native to Korea and China and has been used extensively in eastern Asia. The common name, 'ginseng', is used to describe a number of chemically different species of *Panax*, so caution must be used when interpreting data between species.

Health authorities in Germany and the WHO endorse the use of *P. ginseng* as a tonic or restorative agent for invigoration and fortification in times of fatigue, debility, or physical or mental exhaustion. It does not appear to be effective for hot flushes. Case reports have associated ginseng with post-menopausal bleeding and mastalgia. Interactions have been observed with warfarin, phenelzine and alcohol.

Piper methysticum (kava kava)

In the South Pacific, kava kava has been used for recreational and medicinal purposes for thousands of years. A Cochrane Review concluded that it may be an effective symptomatic treatment for anxiety, but the data about menopausal symptoms are conflicting. Concern about liver damage has led regulatory authorities to suspend or withdraw kava kava.

Other herbs

Wild yam cream, St John's wort, *Agnus castus* (chasteberry), liquorice root and valerian root are also popular, but no good evidence shows that they have any effect on menopausal symptoms. Claims have been made that steroids (diosgenin) in wild yam (*Dioscorea villosa*) can be converted in the body to progesterone, but this is biochemically impossible in man. Some dietary components and herbal products can influence bone metabolism, particularly by inhibiting bone resorption, thus having beneficial effects on the skeleton. Most of the data are limited to *in vitro* or animal models. For example, it has been reported that a number of common vegetables, including onion, garlic and parsley, can inhibit bone resorption in ovariectomized rats. Essential oils derived from sage, rosemary, thyme and other herbs inhibit osteoclast activity *in vitro*.

Botanical drug interactions

Herbal remedies need to be used with caution in women with a contraindication to oestrogen, as some botanicals have oestrogenic properties (soy, red clover, ginseng). Thus, they should not be used by women with a hormone-dependent condition such as breast cancer or endometriosis. They may interact with selective oestrogen receptor modulators (tamoxifen, raloxifene) or aromatase inhibitors (anastrozole, letrozole).

Other consequences of herb–drug interactions include bleeding when combined with warfarin or aspirin; hypertension, coma and mild serotonin syndrome when combined with serotonin reuptake inhibitors; and reduced efficacy of antiepileptics and oral contraceptives. For example, *G. biloba* (ginkgo) can cause bleeding when combined with warfarin or aspirin, high blood pressure when combined with a thiazide diuretic, and even coma when combined with trazodone. *P. ginseng* (ginseng) reduces the blood concentrations of alcohol and warfarin and can induce mania when used concomitantly with phenelzine.

Hypericum perforatum (St John's wort) reduces the blood concentrations of cyclosporin, midazolam, tacrolimus, amitriptyline, digoxin, warfarin and theophylline. Cases have been reported in which reduced concentrations of cyclosporin led to organ rejection. *Hypericum* also causes breakthrough bleeding and unplanned pregnancies when used concomitantly with oral contraceptives. It also causes serotonin syndrome when used in combination with selective serotonin reuptake inhibitors (for example, sertraline and paroxetine).

Homeopathy

Samuel Hahnemann (1755–1843), a German physician and scientist, was the first to enunciate the central tenets of homeopathic philosophy. He believed in a 'vital force' that animates and regulates the human form and directs growth, healing and repair. He postulated that the homeopathic remedy acted through the vital force, stimulating a healing or self-regulating response. He then put forward the principle of 'similars', maintaining that patients with particular signs and symptoms can be cured if given a drug that produces the same signs and symptoms in a healthy individual. He also pursued the concept of minimum dose – the smallest amount of a substance that can be given to avoid side-effects and yet will still bring about a healing response. He found that the curative action of certain preparations seemed to be stronger at some of the lower doses, particularly when shaken vigorously (a process known as succussion), than at higher doses. The mechanisms that underlie the biological response to ultramolecular dilutions, however, are scientifically unclear. Data from case histories, observational studies and a small number of randomized trials are encouraging, but more research clearly is needed.

Dehydroepiandrosterone

Dehydroepiandrosterone (DHEA) is a steroid secreted by the adrenal cortex. It is mostly produced in a sulphated form (DHEA-S), which may be converted to DHEA in many tissues. Blood levels of DHEA decrease dramatically with age. This led to suggestions that the effects of ageing can be counteracted by DHEA 'replacement therapy'. Dehydroepiandrosterone is increasingly being used in the USA, where it is classed as a food supplement, for its supposed anti-ageing effects. Some studies have shown beneficial effects on the skeleton, cognition, wellbeing, libido and the vagina. No evidence shows that DHEA has any effect on hot flashes. The short-term effects of taking DHEA are still controversial, and the possible harmful effects of long-term use are as yet unknown.

Progesterone transdermal creams

Progesterone has been prepared in gels and creams for a number of years. One licensed gel is available in Europe; however, it is indicated for local use on the breast – not for systemic therapy. A vaginal gel for endometrial protection has been studied.

The various transdermal preparations for systemic use usually contain micronized progesterone in concentrations of 0.17–64.0 mg/g, with most products containing about 30.0 mg/g in a cream. Progesterone creams have been advocated for the treatment of menopausal symptoms and skeletal protection. At present, there are insufficient published data to show that transdermal progesterone has a positive effect on vasomotor symptoms or the skeleton. To avoid the side-effects of progestogens, women who take systemic oestrogens may use transdermal progesterone creams for endometrial protection. No consistent evidence, however, shows that transdermal progesterone creams can prevent mitotic activity or induce secretory change in an oestrogen-primed endometrium. Thus, women who use such a combination are increasing their risk of endometrial cancer, and the practice should be discouraged. Further research is needed to establish whether progesterone creams can play a role in the management of the short- and long-term consequences of the menopause.

'Mechanical' therapies

The term 'mechanical' is used, as these therapies do not involve ingestion or application of any agent. They include acupuncture, reflexology, magnetism, acupressure, the Alexander technique, Ayurveda, osteopathy and Reiki. Data with regard to the menopause are scant, and well-designed, adequately powered studies are required.

Acupuncture

Acupuncture is the stimulation of special points on the body, usually by the insertion of fine needles. It originated in the Far East about 2000 years ago, and, in its original form, acupuncture was based on the principles of traditional Chinese medicine (Figure 11.1). According to these, the workings of the human body are controlled by a vital force or energy called 'qi' (pronounced 'chee'), which circulates between the organs along channels called meridians. There are 12 main meridians, and these correspond to 12 major functions or 'organs' of the body. Qi energy must flow in the correct strength and quality through each of these meridians and organs for health to be maintained. The acupuncture points are located along the meridians and provide one means of altering the flow of qi. The evidence from randomized trials that acupuncture helps menopausal symptoms is conflicting.

Reflexology

Reflexology aims to relieve stress or treat health conditions through the application of pressure to specific points or areas of the feet. The underlying idea of reflexology is that areas of the feet correspond to (and affect) other parts of the body (Figure 11.2). In some cases, pressure may also be applied to the hands or ears. Techniques similar to reflexology have been used for thousands of years in Egypt, China and other areas. Although it has been used for various conditions such as pain, anxiety and premenstrual syndrome, few studies have looked at menopausal complaints. Limited data show no improvement of vasomotor symptoms. Thus, currently, its use is uncertain.

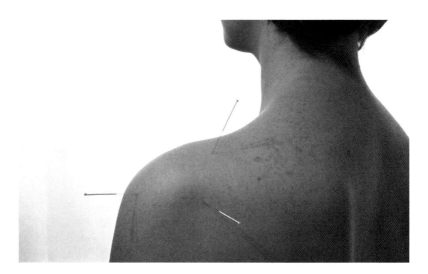

Figure 11.1 Acupuncture needles. Courtesy of British Acupuncture Council

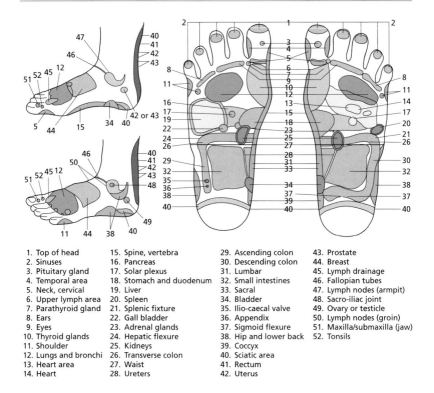

1. Top of head
2. Sinuses
3. Pituitary gland
4. Temporal area
5. Neck, cervical
6. Upper lymph area
7. Parathyroid gland
8. Ears
9. Eyes
10. Thyroid glands
11. Shoulder
12. Lungs and bronchi
13. Heart area
14. Heart

15. Spine, vertebra
16. Pancreas
17. Solar plexus
18. Stomach and duodenum
19. Liver
20. Spleen
21. Splenic fixture
22. Gall bladder
23. Adrenal glands
24. Hepatic flexure
25. Kidneys
26. Transverse colon
27. Waist
28. Ureters

29. Ascending colon
30. Descending colon
31. Lumbar
32. Small intestines
33. Sacral
34. Bladder
35. Ilio-caecal valve
36. Appendix
37. Sigmoid flexure
38. Hip and lower back
39. Coccyx
40. Sciatic area
41. Rectum
42. Uterus

43. Prostate
44. Breast
45. Lymph drainage
46. Fallopian tubes
47. Lymph nodes (armpit)
48. Sacro-iliac joint
49. Ovary or testicle
50. Lymph nodes (groin)
51. Maxilla/submaxilla (jaw)
52. Tonsils

Figure 11.2 Reflexology chart

Magnetism

Magnets are marketed in various forms such as bracelets and insoles. There is no known mechanism of action by which magnet therapies can treat hot flushes. There is no evidence of benefit at present.

Further reading

General

British Menopause Society Council Consensus Statement 2007. Alternative and complementary therapies. www.thebms.org.uk/statementcontent.php?id=2.

Gold EB, Bair Y, Zhang G, *et al*. Cross-sectional analysis of specific complementary and alternative medicine (CAM) use by racial/ethnic group and menopausal status: the Study of Women's Health Across the Nation (SWAN). *Menopause* 2007;**14**:612–23.

MHRA Traditional Herbal Medicines Registration Scheme. www.mhra.gov.uk/ Howweregulate/Medicines/Herbalandhomoeopathicmedicines/Herbalmedicines/ PlacingaherbalmedicineontheUKmarket/TraditionalHerbalMedicinesRegistration Scheme/index.htm.

National Center for Complementary and Alternative Medicine (NCCAM) Menopausal Symptoms and CAM. nccam.nih.gov/health/menopauseandcam.

Nedrow A, Miller J, Walker M, *et al.* Complementary and alternative therapies for the management of menopause-related symptoms: a systematic evidence review. *Arch Intern Med* 2006;**166**:1453–65.

Piersen CE, Booth NL, Sun Y, *et al.* Chemical and biological characterization and clinical evaluation of botanical dietary supplements: a phase I red clover extract as a model. *Curr Med Chem* 2004;**11**:1361–74.

Royal College of Obstetricians and Gynaecologists (RCOG). Alternatives to HRT for the management of symptoms of the menopause. Scientific Advisory Committee Opinion Paper 6. London: RCOG, 2006. www.rcog.org.uk/index.asp? PageID=1561.

Saper RB, Kales SN, Paquin J, *et al.* Heavy metal content of ayurvedic herbal medicine products. *JAMA* 2004;**292**:2868–73.

Thomas K, Coleman P. Use of complementary or alternative medicine in a general population in Great Britain. Results from the National Omnibus survey. *J Public Health (Oxf)* 2004;**26**:152–7.

van der Sluijs CP, Bensoussan A, Liyanage L, Shah S. Women's health during mid-life survey: the use of complementary and alternative medicine by symptomatic women transitioning through menopause in Sydney. *Menopause* 2007;**14**: 397–403.

Yong EL, Wong SP, Shen P, *et al.* Standardization and evaluation of botanical mixtures: lessons from a traditional Chinese herb, Epimedium, with oestrogenic properties. *Novartis Found Symp* 2007;**282**:173–88.

Botanicals

Bai W, Henneicke-von Zepelin HH, Wang S, *et al.* Efficacy and tolerability of a medicinal product containing an isopropanolic black cohosh extract in Chinese women with menopausal symptoms: a randomized, double blind, parallel-controlled study versus tibolone. *Maturitas* 2007;**58**:31–41.

Balk E, Chung M, Chew P, *et al.* Effects of soy on health outcomes. *Evid Rep Technol Assess (Summ)* 2005;**126**:1–8.

Chitturi S, Farrell GC. Hepatotoxic slimming aids and other herbal hepatotoxins. *J Gastroenterol Hepatol* 2008;**23**:366–73.

Coon JT, Pittler MH, Ernst E. Trifolium pratense isoflavones in the treatment of menopausal hot flushes: a systematic review and meta-analysis. *Phytomedicine* 2007;**14**:153–9.

De Smet PA. Clinical risk management of herb–drug interactions. *Br J Clin Pharmacol* 2007;**63**:258–67.

Dodin S, Lemay A, Jacques H, *et al*. The effects of flaxseed dietary supplement on lipid profile, bone mineral density, and symptoms in menopausal women: a randomized, double-blind, wheat germ placebo-controlled clinical trial. *J Clin Endocrinol Metab* 2005;**90**:1390–7.

Heyerick A, Vervarcke S, Depypere H, *et al*. A first prospective, randomized, double-blind, placebo-controlled study on the use of a standardized hop extract to alleviate menopausal discomforts. *Maturitas* 2006;**54**:164–75.

Howes LG, Howes JB, Knight DC. Isoflavone therapy for menopausal flushes: a systematic review and meta-analysis. *Maturitas* 2006;**55**:203–11.

Hu Z, Yang X, Ho PC, *et al*. Herb–drug interactions: a literature review. *Drugs* 2005;**65**:1239–82.

ISOHEART. www.isoheart.kvl.dk.

Komesaroff PA, Black CVS, Cable V, Sudhir K. Effects of wild yam extract on menopausal symptoms, lipids and sex hormones in healthy menopausal women. *Climacteric* 2001;**4**:144–50.

Kupfersztain C, Rotem C, Fagot R, Kaplan B. The immediate effect of natural plant extract, *Angelica sinensis* and *Matricaria chamomilla* (Climex) for the treatment of hot flushes during menopause. A preliminary report. *Clin Exp Obstet Gynecol* 2003;**30**:203–6.

Kwee SH, Tan HH, Marsman A, Wauters C. The effect of Chinese herbal medicines (CHM) on menopausal symptoms compared to hormone replacement therapy (HRT) and placebo. *Maturitas* 2007;**58**:83–90.

Lethaby AE, Brown J, Marjoribanks J, *et al*. Phytoestrogens for vasomotor menopausal symptoms. *Cochrane Database Syst Rev* 2007;**4**:CD001395.

Low Dog T. Menopause: a review of botanical dietary supplements. *Am J Med* 2005;**118**(Suppl 12B):98–108.

Meijerman I, Beijnen JH, Schellens JH. Herb–drug interactions in oncology: focus on mechanisms of induction. *Oncologist* 2006;**11**:742–52.

Messina M, McCaskill-Stevens W, Lampe JW. Addressing the soy and breast cancer relationship: review, commentary, and workshop proceedings. *J Natl Cancer Inst* 2006;**98**:1275–84.

Newton KM, Reed SD, LaCroix AZ, *et al*. Treatment of vasomotor symptoms of menopause with black cohosh, multibotanicals, soy, hormone therapy, or placebo: a randomized trial. *Ann Intern Med* 2006;**145**:869–79.

Nortier JL, Vanherweghem JL. Renal interstitial fibrosis and urothelial carcinoma associated with the use of a Chinese herb (*Aristolochia fangchi*). *Toxicology* 2002;**181–182**:577–80.

Palacios S, Pornel B, Bergeron C, *et al*. Endometrial safety assessment of a specific and standardized soy extract according to international guidelines. *Menopause* 2007;**14**:1006–11.

PHYTOPREVENT. www.phytocancereu.com/index.html/

The Prevention of Osteoporosis by Nutritional Phytoestrogens (PHYTOS). ec.europa.eu/research/endocrine/pdf/qlk1-ct2000–00431-year1.pdf.

Pockaj BA, Gallagher JG, Loprinzi CL, *et al*. Phase III double-blind, randomized, placebo-controlled crossover trial of black cohosh in the management of hot flashes: NCCTG Trial N01CC1. *J Clin Oncol* 2006;**24**:2836–41.

Pruthi S, Thompson SL, Novotny PJ, *et al*. Pilot evaluation of flaxseed for the management of hot flashes. *J Soc Integr Oncol* 2007;5:106–12.

Putnam SE, Scutt AM, Bicknell K, *et al*. Natural products as alternative treatments for metabolic bone disorders and for maintenance of bone health. *Phytother Res* 2007;21:99–112.

Reed SD, Newton KM, LaCroix AZ, *et al*. Vaginal, endometrial, and reproductive hormone findings: randomized, placebo-controlled trial of black cohosh, multibotanical herbs, and dietary soy for vasomotor symptoms: the Herbal Alternatives for Menopause (HALT) Study. *Menopause* 2008;15:51–8.

Rowland IR, Wiseman H, Sanders TA, *et al*. Interindividual variation in metabolism of soy isoflavones and lignans: influence of habitual diet on equol production by the gut microflora. *Nutr Cancer* 2000;36:27–32.

Sacks FM, Lichtenstein A, Van Horn L, *et al*.; American Heart Association Nutrition Committee. Soy protein, isoflavones, and cardiovascular health: an American Heart Association Science Advisory for professionals from the Nutrition Committee. *Circulation* 2006;113:1034–44.

Taylor DM, Walsham N, Taylor SE, Wong L. Potential interactions between prescription drugs and complementary and alternative medicines among patients in the emergency department. *Pharmacotherapy* 2006;26:634–40.

Tice JA, Ettinger B, Ensrud K, *et al*. Phytoestrogen supplements for the treatment of hot flashes: the Isoflavone Clover Extract (ICE) Study: a randomized controlled trial. *JAMA* 2003;290:207–14.

Van de Weijer PHM, Barentsen R. Isoflavones from red clover (Promensil®) significantly reduce menopausal hot flush symptoms compared with placebo. *Maturitas* 2002;42:187–93.

Winther K, Rein E, Hedman C. Femal, a herbal remedy made from pollen extracts, reduces hot flushes and improves quality of life in menopausal women: a randomized, placebo-controlled, parallel study. *Climacteric* 2005;8:162–70.

Zhou SF, Zhou ZW, Li CG, *et al*. Identification of drugs that interact with herbs in drug development. *Drug Discov Today* 2007;12:664–73.

Homeopathy

Bordet MF, Colas A, Marijnen P, *et al*. Treating hot flushes in menopausal women with homeopathic treatment – results of an observational study. *Homeopathy* 2008;97:10–15.

Jacobs J, Herman P, Heron K, *et al*. Homeopathy for menopausal symptoms in breast cancer survivors: a preliminary randomized controlled trial. *J Altern Complement Med* 2005;11:21–7.

Milgrom LR. Is homeopathy possible? *J R Soc Health* 2006;126:211–18.

Thompson EA, Montgomery A, Douglas D, Reilly D. A pilot, randomized, double-blinded, placebo-controlled trial of individualized homeopathy for symptoms of estrogen withdrawal in breast-cancer survivors. *J Altern Complement Med* 2005;11:13–20.

Dehydroepiandrosterone

Grimley Evans J, Malouf R, Huppert F, van Niekerk JK. Dehydroepiandrosterone (DHEA) supplementation for cognitive function in healthy elderly people. *Cochrane Database Syst Rev* 2006;4:CD006221.

Panjari M, Davis SR. DHEA therapy for women: effect on sexual function and wellbeing. *Hum Reprod Update* 2007;13:239–48.

Raven PW, Hinson JP. Dehydroepiandrosterone (DHEA) and the menopause: an update. *Menopause Int* 2007;13:75–8.

von Mühlen D, Laughlin GA, Kritz-Silverstein D, Barrett-Connor E. The Dehydroepiandrosterone And WellNess (DAWN) study: research design and methods. *Contemp Clin Trials* 2007;28:153–68.

Progesterone transdermal creams

Leonetti HB, Longo S, Anasti JN. Transdermal progesterone cream for vasomotor symptoms and postmenopausal bone loss. *Obstet Gynecol* 1999;94:225–8.

Lydeking-Olsen E, Beck-Jensen JE, Setchell KD, Holm-Jensen T. Soymilk or progesterone for prevention of bone loss – a 2 year randomized, placebo-controlled trial. *Eur J Nutr* 2004;43:246–57.

Vashisht A, Wadsworth F, Carey A, *et al*. Bleeding profiles and effects on the endometrium for women using a novel combination of transdermal oestradiol and natural progesterone cream as part of a continuous combined hormone replacement regime. *BJOG* 2005;112:1402–6.

Wren BG, Champion SM, Willetts K, *et al*. Transdermal progesterone and its effect on vasomotor symptoms, blood lipid levels, bone metabolic markers, moods, and quality of life for postmenopausal women. *Menopause* 2003;10:13–18.

'Mechanical' therapies

Avis NE, Legault C, Coeytaux RR, *et al*. A randomized, controlled pilot study of acupuncture treatment for menopausal hot flashes. *Menopause* 2008;15:1070–8.

Carpenter JS, Neal JG. Other complementary and alternative medicine modalities: acupuncture, magnets, reflexology, and homeopathy. *Am J Med* 2005;118(Suppl 12B):109–17.

Deng G, Vickers A, Yeung S, *et al*. Randomized, controlled trial of acupuncture for the treatment of hot flashes in breast cancer patients. *J Clin Oncol* 2007;25:5584–90.

Frisk J, Carlhäll S, Källström AC, *et al*. Long-term follow-up of acupuncture and hormone therapy on hot flushes in women with breast cancer: a prospective, randomized, controlled multicenter trial. *Climacteric* 2008;11:166–74.

Mandrekar JN, Cha SS, Zais T, *et al*. Acupuncture for hot flashes: a randomized, sham-controlled clinical study. *Menopause* 2007;14:45–52.

Nedstrand E, Wyon Y, Hammar M, Wijma K. Psychological well-being improves in women with breast cancer after treatment with applied relaxation or electro-acupuncture for vasomotor symptom. *J Psychosom Obstet Gynaecol* 2006;27: 193–9.

Nir Y, Huang MI, Schnyer R, *et al.* Acupuncture for postmenopausal hot flashes. *Maturitas* 2007;**56**:383–95.

Williamson J, White A, Hart A, Ernst E. Randomised controlled trial of reflexology for menopausal symptoms. *BJOG* 2002;**109**:1050–5.

Zaborowska E, Brynhildsen J, Damberg S, *et al.* Effects of acupuncture, applied relaxation, estrogens and placebo on hot flushes in postmenopausal women: an analysis of two prospective, parallel, randomized studies. *Climacteric* 2007;**10**:38–45.

WOMEN WITH SPECIAL NEEDS

12 Premature ovarian failure

Introduction

The terms 'premature ovarian failure' (POF) and 'premature menopause' are often used interchangeably, although there is debate about which term is best. Some women with POF present with oligomenorrhoea and have persistent sporadic ovarian activity. Menopause implies permanent cessation of ovarian activity and menstruation. Ideally, premature menopause should be defined as menopause that occurs at an age more than two standard deviations below the mean estimated for the reference population. In the absence of reliable estimates of age of natural menopause in developing countries, the age of 40 years is used frequently as an arbitrary limit below which the menopause is said to be premature. In the developed world, however, the age of 45 years should be taken as the cut-off point.

The condition is common. Overall, POF is responsible for 4–18% of cases of secondary amenorrhoea and 10–28% of primary amenorrhoea. It is estimated to affect 1% of women younger than 40 years and 0.1% of those under 30 years.

Aetiology

Primary premature ovarian failure

Primary POF can occur at any age, even in teenagers. It can present as primary or secondary amenorrhoea or oligomenorrhoea. Even in the presence of ovarian failure, some women may have continuing erratic spontaneous ovarian activity and have further periods which may be irregular and unpredictable. Moreover, while a woman with POF has a greatly reduced chance of spontaneous pregnancy, it is still possible.

In the great majority of cases of POF, no cause is found. Traditional texts have concentrated on describing ovarian failure as being associated with a deficient number of primordial follicles from the onset of menarche, accelerated follicle atresia or follicles resistant to stimulation by gonadotrophins. In the absence of a non-invasive test to distinguish between follicular depletion or dysfunction, the only alternative is laparoscopic ovarian biopsy. The validity of single biopsies has been questioned, pregnancies occurring despite histological lack of follicles in the biopsy material. The causes are detailed in Box 12.1.

Chromosome abnormalities

The requirement for two intact X chromosomes for normal follicular development was determined in the 1960s. A critical region on the X-chromosome (POF1), which ranges from Xq13 to Xq26, that relates to normal ovarian function has been identified, as has a second gene of paternal origin (POF2), which is located at Xq13.3–q21.1. Idiopathic POF can be familial or sporadic, and the familial pattern of inheritance is compatible with X-linked inheritance (with incomplete penetrance) or an autosomal dominant mode of inheritance. In Turner syndrome, complete absence of one X chromosome (45XO) results in ovarian dysgenesis and primary ovarian failure. Familial POF has been linked with fragile X permutations. Fragile X mutations occur at least 10 times more often in women with POF than the general population. Women with Down's syndrome (trisomy 21) also have early menopause. The BEPS syndrome is a rare autosomal dominant condition that leads to congenital abnormalities of the eye, including blepharophimosis, ptosis and epicanthus inversis. In BEPS I, eyelid malformation cosegregates with POF and has been mapped to chromosome 3q.17.

Box 12.1

Causes of premature ovarian failure

Primary
Chromosome abnormalities
Follicle-stimulating hormone receptor gene polymorphism and inhibin B
   mutation
Enzyme deficiencies
Autoimmune disease

Secondary
Chemotherapy and radiotherapy
Bilateral oophorectomy or surgical menopause
Hysterectomy without oophorectomy/uterine artery embolization
Infection

Follicle-stimulating hormone receptor gene polymorphism and inhibin B mutation

Resistance to the action of gonadotrophins can lead to the clinical features of POF, and this has been shown in a cohort of Finnish families. This is a very rare cause. In addition, a mutation in the inhibin gene (see Chapter 1) that has a frequency 10-fold higher than in control patients (7% versus 0.7%) has been identified. These patients experienced ovarian failure at an early age – often before the second decade of life.

Enzyme deficiencies

A number of enzyme deficiencies have been found to be associated with increased risk of POF. The most common of these is the autosomal recessive condition of galactosaemia, in which there is a deficiency in the enzyme galactose-1-phosphate uridyltransferase. Accumulation of galactose results in damage to the liver, eyes and kidneys. It increases the risk of POF, although spontaneous pregnancy can occur. The cause seems to be a galactose-induced reduction in total germ-cell development during oogenesis. Other proposed mechanisms include accelerated follicular atresia and biologically inactive isoforms of follicle-stimulating hormone (FSH). Other enzyme abnormalities associated with POF include deficiencies of 17α-hydroxylase, 17–20 desmolase and cholesterol desmolase. Deficiency of 17α-hydroxylase can prevent oestradiol synthesis, leading to primary amenorrhoea and elevated levels of gonadotrophins, even though developing follicles are present.

Patients with a deficiency of cholesterol desmolase are not able to produce biologically active steroids and rarely survive to adulthood.

Autoimmune disease

Premature ovarian failure is frequently associated with autoimmune disorders, particularly hypothyroidism (25%), Addison's disease (3%) and diabetes mellitus (2.5%). Other coexisting conditions may include Crohn's disease, vitiligo, pernicious anaemia, systemic lupus erythematosus or rheumatoid arthritis. Addison's disease may be present as part of a polyglandular failure syndrome. The type I syndrome, which is associated with adrenal failure, hypoparathyroidism and chronic mucocutaneous candidiasis, and mainly occurs in children, is associated with POF. The type II syndrome may present much later with hypothyroidism and is less consistently associated with POF.

The prevalence of antibodies directed against the ovary has been the subject of significant research. Circulating anti-ovarian antibodies have been found in 10–69% of women with POF but also in a significant number of controls. Anti-gonadotrophin receptor antibodies have been isolated, but their significance remains unclear. Antibodies against steroid-producing cells have proved most promising in terms of predicting which patients may develop ovarian failure as part of the polyglandular syndrome; however, these women constitute a minority of those with POF.

Secondary premature ovarian failure

Secondary POF is becoming more important as survival after the treatment of malignancy continues to improve. The development of techniques to conserve ovarian tissue or oocytes before therapy is instigated, however, should help with maintenance of fertility. The causes of secondary POF are detailed below. Currently, there is no evidence that ovarian stimulation for *in vitro* fertilization advances the age of the menopause.

Chemotherapy and radiotherapy

The likelihood of ovarian failure after chemotherapy or radiotherapy depends on the agent used, dosage levels, interval between treatments and, particularly, the age of the patient, probably reflecting the age-related progressive natural decline in the oocyte pool. The prepubertal ovary is relatively resistant to the effects of chemotherapeutic alkylating agents. The use of gonadotrophin hormone-releasing analogues to suppress ovarian activity in order to mimic this protection is as yet not supported by randomized, controlled trials.

Radiation-induced ovarian failure usually results in sterility when the total dose exceeds 6 Gy. As with chemotherapy, however, prepubertal girls are more resistant to irradiation. Normal menstruation after treatment does not necessarily mean the ovaries are unaffected, and premature menopause can occur, resulting in a shorter reproductive span. Surgical transposition of the ovaries outside the direct field of treatment has been described. A successful term pregnancy also depends on a normal uterine environment that is not only receptive to implantation but also able to accommodate normal growth of the fetus. The degree of damage to the uterus depends on the total dose of radiation and the site of irradiation. The prepubertal uterus is more vulnerable to the effects of pelvic irradiation, with doses of radiation of 14–30 Gy likely to result in uterine dysfunction. High-dose pelvic radiotherapy in young women will have long-term effects on the uterine vasculature and development. Adverse pregnancy outcomes have been described for women treated with total body irradiation, and include increased risk of early pregnancy loss, preterm birth, and delivery of infants with low or very low birthweight. An excess risk of infants of low birthweight and preterm birth also exists among mothers who received abdominal irradiation for Wilms' tumour in childhood.

Bilateral oophorectomy or surgical menopause

Bilateral oophorectomy results in immediate menopause, which may be intensely symptomatic. The implications of this procedure require detailed discussion with the patient in view of the increased morbidity and mortality in those who cannot, or will not, take oestrogen replacement.

Hysterectomy without oophorectomy/uterine artery embolization

Both procedures can diminish ovarian reserve and lead to ovarian failure. Uterine artery embolization is a technique used for fibroids. The diagnosis of POF in hysterectomized women may be difficult, as not all have acute symptoms, and in the absence of a uterus, the pointer of amenorrhoea is absent. A case could be made for annual estimates of levels of FSH in women who have had a hysterectomy/uterine artery embolization before the age of 40 years.

Infection

Tuberculosis and mumps are infections that have been implicated most commonly. The increasing incidence of tuberculosis and the emergence of multi-drug resistant strains of bacilli is of concern. In most cases, normal ovarian function returns after infection with mumps. Malaria, varicella and shigella infections have also been implicated in POF.

Presentation and assessment

The most common presentation is secondary amenorrhoea or oligomenorrhoea in a woman younger than 40 years, which may be accompanied by hot flushes. Use of combined oestrogen and progestogen or long-acting depot contraceptives results in a proportion of women who present with persistent amenorrhoea when these forms of contraception are stopped. POF may be diagnosed in women seeking treatment for infertility.

Coexisting disease must be detected, particularly hypothyroidism, Addison's disease, diabetes mellitus and any chromosome abnormalities in women with primary ovarian failure – especially those who have not achieved successful pregnancy (Box 12.2). The diagnostic usefulness of ovarian biopsy outside the context of a research setting has yet to be proved.

Consequences of oestrogen deficiency

Women with untreated premature menopause are at increased risk of developing osteoporosis, cardiovascular disease, cognitive decline, dementia and parkinsonism but at lower risk of breast malignancy. Mean life expectancy in women with menopause before the age of 40 years is 2.0 years shorter than

---

Box 12.2

Investigation of premature menopause

- Estimates of follicle-stimulating hormone (×2)
- Thyroid function tests
- Autoimmune screen for polyendocrinopathy
- Chromosome analysis (with screening for Fragile X), especially in women younger than 30 years
- Estimates of bone mineral density through dual X-ray absorptiometry (DXA) (optional)
- Adrenocorticotrophic hormone stimulation test if Addison's disease is suspected (optional)

---

that in women with menopause after the age of 55 years. Premature menopause can lead to reduced peak bone mass (if the women is younger than 25 years) or early bone loss thereafter. The increased risk of coronary heart disease has been noted, especially in smokers. Thus, women contemplating oophorectomy before the age of 40 should be advised of the consequences of oestrogen deficiency.

Management

Counselling

Patients must be provided with adequate information. Women may find it a difficult diagnosis to accept, especially if they wish to have children. National and international support groups for POF exist, and these provide helpful psychological support for many women. Women need to be aware that, in the absence of bilateral oophorectomy, ovulation may occur again, often intermittently, and cyclical menstrual bleeding or even spontaneous pregnancy can result.

Hormone replacement therapy

Oestrogen replacement therapy is the mainstay of treatment for women with POF and is recommended until the average age of natural menopause (52 years in the UK) (Chapter 1). This view is endorsed by regulatory bodies such as the Committee on Safety of Medicines in the UK. No evidence shows that oestrogen replacement increases the risk of breast cancer to a level greater than that found in normally menstruating women, and women with POF do not need to start mammographic screening early. Hormone replacement therapy (HRT) or the combined oestrogen and progestogen contraceptive pill may be used. No clinical trial evidence attests the efficacy or safety of the use of non-oestrogen-based treatments, such as bisphosphonates, strontium ranelate or raloxifene, in these women (see Chapter 9). The evidence of safety of bisphosphonates or strontium ranelate on the developing fetal skeleton is unknown.

A commonly adopted form of treatment is the combined oral contraceptive pill. The latter has the psychological benefit of being a treatment used by many of the patient's peer group. There is a paucity of controlled trial data on how to base treatment decisions. The only direct comparison of ethinyloestradiol and conjugated equine oestrogen is a study of 17 women with Turner syndrome. In this short study, no difference was seen between the two oestrogens with respect to effect on the endometrium, hyperinsulinaemia or lipid profile. Ethinyloestradiol had a more potent effect on markers of bone turnover and suppression of gonadotrophins. Women with POF who take HRT may need a higher dose of oestrogen to control vasomotor symptoms than women in their 50s.

Some patients report reduced libido or sexual function despite apparently adequate doses of oestrogen replacement. This may be more common in oophorectomized women, and consideration should be given to additional treatment with testosterone. This may be administered with either patches or subcutaneous implants (see Chapter 6).

Fertility and contraception

It is important to ascertain whether the woman wishes to have children or not. While women with premature menopause have traditionally been considered to be infertile, the lifetime chance of spontaneous conception in women with karyotypically normal POF has been estimated at 5–15%, with the age of the patient at the time of diagnosis being an important determinant. A number of ovarian reserve tests (ORTs) have been designed to determine oocyte reserve and quality. These include early-follicular-phase blood values of FSH, oestradiol, inhibin B and anti-Müllerian hormone (AMH); the antral follicle count (AFC); the ovarian volume (OVVOL); and the ovarian blood flow, as well as the clomiphene citrate challenge test (CCCT), the exogenous FSH ORT (EFORT), and the gonadotrophin agonist stimulation test (GAST). A systematic review of ORTs has shown that they have only modest-to-poor predictive properties.

Donor oocyte *in vitro* fertilization (IVF) is the treatment of choice for women with primary and secondary POF. Women with spontaneous, karyotypically normal POF have similar success rates to women who undergo conventional IVF. Patients can be reassured that there is no urgency for treatment after a diagnosis of POF. The age of the oocyte rather than the age of the recipient determines the chance of success. The use of a sibling's oocyte may decrease the likelihood of pregnancy.

Oocyte donation is also an option for women with Turner syndrome, and pregnancy rates in observational studies are similar to those with oocyte donation for other indications. The risk of miscarriage, however, is greater. Cardiovascular and other complications, such as hypertension and pre-eclampsia, occur more frequently in women with Turner syndrome, and it has been suggested that embryo transfer be limited to a single embryo to avoid additional complications as a result of multiple pregnancies. Pretreatment screening to detect previously undiagnosed maternal congenital cardiac abnormalities is essential.

In women having chemotherapy or radiotherapy, IVF with embryo freezing prior to treatment currently offers the highest likelihood of a future pregnancy should they experience POF as a result of their treatment. However, this depends on having a partner with whom the woman wishes to have a family. Recent technical advances in oocyte preservation have improved live birth rates after freezing of mature eggs. It is still less successful than embryo freezing. Ovulation induction risks delaying treatment in those with aggressive tumours, and in women with hormone-sensitive tumours, such as breast cancer, there is the additional concern of the safety of ovarian stimulation. Cryopreservation of ovarian tissue is still largely experimental, although pregnancies have been reported. This technique would be an option for prepubertal girls where ovulation induction is not possible.

Women who do not wish to have children need to consider using an effective form of contraception. The next decision will be how long contraception should be continued. Traditionally, women have been advised that contraception can be stopped if they have been amenorrhoeic for 2 years before the age of 50 years and one year above that. However, the menstrual pattern is difficult to establish in HRT users, and one may advise using contraception until the age of 55 years.

Further reading

Aetiology

Birch JM, Pang D, Alston RD, *et al.* Survival from cancer in teenagers and young adults in England, 1979–2003. *Br J Cancer* 2008;**99**:830–5.

Elder K, Mathews T, Kutner E, *et al.* Impact of gonadotrophin stimulation for assisted reproductive technology on ovarian ageing and menopause. *Reprod BioMed Online* 2008;**16**:611–16.

ESHRE Capri Workshop Group. Genetic aspects of female reproduction. *Hum Reprod Update* 2008;**14**:293–307.

Gubbels CS, Land JA, Rubio-Gozalbo ME. Fertility and impact of pregnancies on the mother and child in classic galactosemia. *Obstet Gynecol Surv* 2008;**63**:334–43.

Halmesmäki KH, Hurskainen RA, Cacciatore B, *et al*. Effect of hysterectomy or LNG-IUS on serum inhibin B levels and ovarian blood flow. *Maturitas* 2007;**57**:279–85.

Hehenkamp WJ, Volkers NA, Broekmans FJ, *et al*. Loss of ovarian reserve after uterine artery embolization: a randomized comparison with hysterectomy. *Hum Reprod* 2007;**22**:1996–2005.

Laml T, Preyer O, Umek W, *et al*. Genetic disorders in premature ovarian failure. *Hum Reprod Update* 2002;**8**:483–91.

Oktay K, Sönmezer M, Oktem O, *et al*. Absence of conclusive evidence for the safety and efficacy of gonadotropin-releasing hormone analogue treatment in protecting against chemotherapy-induced gonadal injury. *Oncologist* 2007;**12**:1055–66.

Pal L, Santoro N. Premature ovarian failure (POF): discordance between somatic and reproductive aging. *Ageing Res Rev* 2002;**1**:413–23.

Wallace WH, Thomson AB, Saran F, Kelsey TW. Predicting age of ovarian failure after radiation to a field that includes the ovaries. *Int J Radiat Oncol Biol Phys* 2005;**62**: 738–44.

Consequences of premature menopause

Atsma F, Bartelink ML, Grobbee DE, van der Schouw YT. Postmenopausal status and early menopause as independent risk factors for cardiovascular disease: a meta-analysis. *Menopause* 2006;**13**:265–79.

Ossewaarde ME, Bots ML, Verbeek AL, *et al*. Age at menopause, cause-specific mortality and total life expectancy. *Epidemiology* 2005;**16**:556–62.

Shuster LT, Gostout BS, Grossardt BR, Rocca WA. Prophylactic oophorectomy in pre-menopausal women and long term health – a review. *Menopause Int* 2008;**14**: 111–16.

Titus-Ernstoff L, Longnecker MP, Newcomb PA, *et al*. Menstrual factors in relation to breast cancer risk. *Cancer Epidemiol Biomarkers Prev* 1998;**7**:783–9.

van der Klift M, de Laet CE, McCloskey EV, *et al*. Risk factors for incident vertebral fractures in men and women: the Rotterdam Study. *J Bone Miner Res* 2004;**19**: 1172–80.

van Der Voort DJ, van Der Weijer PH, Barentsen R. Early menopause: increased fracture risk at older age. *Osteoporos Int* 2003;**14**:525–30.

Management

Broekmans FJ, Kwee J, Hendriks DJ, *et al*. A systematic review of tests predicting ovarian reserve and IVF outcome. *Hum Reprod Update* 2006;**12**:685–718.

Ewertz M, Mellemkjaer L, Poulsen AH, *et al*. Hormone use for menopausal symptoms and risk of breast cancer. A Danish cohort study. *Br J Cancer* 2005;**92**:1293–7.

Faculty of Family Planning and Reproductive Health Care. Clinical Effectiveness Unit. Contraception for women aged over 40 years. *J Fam Plann Reprod Health Care* 2005;**31**:51–64.

Guttman H, Weiner Z, Nikolski E, *et al.* Choosing an oestrogen replacement therapy in young adult women with Turner syndrome. *Clin Endocrinol* 2001;54:159–64.

Hjerrild BE, Mortensen KH, Gravholt CH. Turner syndrome and clinical treatment. *Br Med Bull* 2008;86:77–93.

Kingsberg S. Testosterone treatment for hypoactive sexual desire disorder in post-menopausal women. *J Sex Med* 2007;4(Suppl 3):227–34.

Lee SJ, Schover LR, Partridge AH, *et al.*; American Society of Clinical Oncology. American Society of Clinical Oncology recommendations on fertility preservation in cancer patients. *J Clin Oncol* 2006;24:2917–31.

Løkkegaard E, Jovanovic Z, Heitmann BL, *et al.* The association between early menopause and risk of ischaemic heart disease: influence of hormone therapy. *Maturitas* 2006;53:226–33.

National Collaborating Centre for Women's and Children's Health. *Fertility: Assessment and Treatment for People with Fertility Problems.* London: RCOG Press, 2004:126–7.

Nelson LM, Covington SN, Rebar RW. An update: spontaneous premature ovarian failure is not an early menopause. *Fertil Steril* 2005;83:1327–32.

National Institute of Child Health and Human Development (NICHD). Premature ovarian failure. www.nichd.nih.gov/health/topics/Premature_Ovarian_Failure. cfm.

Pitkin J, Rees MC, Gray S, *et al.* Management of premature menopause. *Menopause Int* 2007;13:44–5.

Silber SJ, Lenahan KM, Levine DJ, *et al.* Ovarian transplantation between monozygotic twins discordant for premature ovarian failure. *N Engl J Med* 2005;353: 58–63.

Stern CJ, Toledo MG, Gook DA, Seymour JF. Fertility preservation in female oncology patients. *Aust N Z J Obstet Gynaecol* 2006;46:15–23.

Sung L, Bustillo M, Mukherjee T, *et al.* Sisters of women with premature ovarian failure may not be ideal ovum donors. *Fertil Steril* 1997;67:912–16.

Tucker D. Premature ovarian failure. In: Rees M, Hope S, Ravnikar V, eds. *The Abnormal Menstrual Cycle.* Abingdon: Taylor and Francis, 2005:111–22.

Ventura JL, Fitzgerald OR, Koziol DE, *et al.* Functional well-being is positively correlated with spiritual well-being in women who have spontaneous premature ovarian failure. *Fertil Steril* 2007;87:584–90.

13 Women with benign medical problems

> Pelvic disorders
> Cardiovascular disease
> Obesity
> Metabolic syndrome
> Endocrine disease
> Neurological disease
> Urinary problems
> Gastrointestinal conditions
> Connective tissue disease
> Other disorders
> Further reading

Some pre-existing medical problems require very careful evaluation by health professionals. While some are relative contraindications to oestrogen, the majority are not. Both oestrogen- and non-oestrogen-based therapies are discussed.

Pelvic disorders

Fibroids

Fibroids (leiomyomas) are oestrogen-dependent tumours that tend to shrink after the menopause. These may become enlarged with oestrogen treatment and cause heavy or painful withdrawal bleeds. The evidence of the effect of different types of hormone replacement therapy (HRT), including tibolone, on fibroid growth is poor. Ultrasound examinations may be helpful in documenting the fibroids, and, if clinically indicated, regular pelvic examinations are recommended. Limited data suggest that raloxifene shrinks fibroids.

Endometriosis

This condition can present a difficult management problem, as oestrogen treatment can theoretically reactivate the disease, even when the patient has had apparent surgical removal of all the endometriotic tissue. Concerns are disease recurrence and malignant changes arising from the presence of residual endometriosis. The risks, however, seem to be small, and the evidence base of various strategies is poor. Patients with a history of endometriosis may be at particular risk of the long-term consequences of oestrogen deficiency as a consequence of repeated courses of gonadotrophin hormone-releasing analogues or bilateral oophorectomy. However, the data are limited. Some gynaecologists avoid starting oestrogen-based HRT for the first 6 months after oophorectomy, preferring to give a progestogen alone, continuous combined therapy or tibolone to control vasomotor symptoms when the patient has extensive disease. No good evidence base is available on whether to recommend an unopposed regimen, an opposed continuous combined regimen or tibolone. Management of potential recurrence is best monitored by responding to the recurrence of symptoms. Data with regard to raloxifene are scant.

Cardiovascular disease

Hypertension

No evidence shows that oestradiol-based HRT increases blood pressure or has an adverse effect in women with pre-existing hypertension. HRT can be taken alongside antihypertensive treatment. Transdermal oestrogen has less effect on the renin-angiotensin system than oral therapy. Rarely, conjugated equine oestrogens may cause severe hypertension that returns to normal when treatment is stopped. Data from trials of tibolone and raloxifene do not show an adverse effect on blood pressure.

Valvular heart disease

Hormone replacement therapy is not contraindicated in women with valvular heart disease. Women who take anticoagulants may have more problems with irregular or heavy bleeding, which requires an adjustment of the dose of progestogen relative to that of the oestrogen. Endometrial biopsy, if required, may need antibiotic cover, but guidelines worldwide vary.

Hyperlipidaemia

In women, the most significant lipid risk factors are high-density lipoprotein C (HDL-C), triglyceride and lipoprotein(a). The increased risk associated with increased levels of triglycerides and low-density lipoprotein C (LDL-C) can be offset by increased levels of HDL. In terms of lipids, the ideal HRT would increase HDL-C without increasing triglyceride and decrease LDL-C and lipoprotein(a). The effects depend on the type of steroid and the route of administration. Oral oestrogen reduces lipoprotein(a) and LDL-C and increases HDL-C and triglycerides. The transdermal route is less effective at reducing lipoprotein(a) and LDL-C but does not increase triglycerides or HDL-C. The type of progestogen is also important. Oral HRT with a non-androgenic progestogen increases HDL-C and triglycerides and decreases LDL-C and lipoprotein(a). Oral HRT with a 19-nortestosterone derivative decreases LDL-C and lipoprotein(a) but does not increase HDL and is neutral for triglycerides. Thus, HRT in these women needs to be tailored to their lipid profile: for example, in women with hypertriglyceridaemia, the transdermal route is preferred to the oral route (Table 13.1). Hormone replacement therapy can be combined with statins.

Raloxifene and tamoxifen reduce levels of total cholesterol and LDL-C while remaining neutral to triglyceride and HDL-C. However, a large, randomized trial (RUTH) found that raloxifene did not reduce the risk of coronary heart disease (CHD). While tibolone does not increase the risk of CHD in osteoporatic women aged 60–85 years, no data exist on tibolone in those with hypertriglyceridaemia (see Chapter 7).

Venous thromboembolism

When taking the history, it is essential to assess the family history, the severity of any personal event, and whether or not it was confirmed objectively. It can be difficult to know whether or not a history of venous thromboembolism (VTE) – sometimes more than 20 years earlier – was a confirmed episode. When in doubt, if a patient was anticoagulated at the time, it is prudent to consider the event confirmed.

Table 13.1

Effects of hormones on lipids

Hormone	Lipid			
	HDL	LDL	Triglyceride	Lipoprotein(a)
Ideal HRT	↑↑	↓↓	↓↓	↓↓
Oral oestrogen	↑	↓↓	↑	↓↓
Transdermal oestrogen	–	↓	↓	↓
Oral progesterone-derived progestogen	↑	↓	↑	↓
Oral testosterone-derived progestogen	–	↓	↓	↓
Tibolone	↓	↓	↓↓	↓
Raloxifene	–	↓	–	↓

↑ Small increase; ↓ small decrease; ↑↑ large increase; ↓↓ large decrease
HDL: high-density lipoprotein; LDL: low-density lipoprotein
– No effect

Women with a personal history of thrombosis

A history of VTE is the biggest risk factor for future VTE and is a relative contraindication to HRT. After a single episode of VTE, a constant risk of recurrence of 5% per year exists when anticoagulation is discontinued.

However, it might be felt in some cases that the risk is outweighed by the benefits of HRT. A thrombophilia screen may then be justified, as the finding of a severe defect or a combination of defects might alter the perceived risk–benefit assessment. A negative thrombophilia screen must not be used to give false reassurance. The woman may be at high risk even though no pathological explanation is present. Women older than 50 years with a history of VTE within the previous year, in addition to thrombophilia screening, should be screened for underlying disease, including malignancy and connective tissue disorders.

If a decision to use HRT is made, the transdermal route is probably safer than oral therapy. Moreover, there may be differences with regard to progestogens in that norpregnane derivatives may be thrombogenic, whereas micronized progesterone and pregnane derivatives do not increase risk.

Occasionally, it is suggested that a woman be anticoagulated to allow HRT to be given. It has to be appreciated that about one in 400 patients on warfarin bleed to death each year, so this is rarely the best option. As raloxifene and progestogens in doses higher than those used for contraceptive purposes increase the risk of VTE, these probably are best avoided (see above and Chapters 8 and 9). No data are available for tibolone in this situation.

Women with family history of thrombosis

To test women with family history of thrombosis for hereditary thrombophilia is only fully informative if a family study is performed. Without a family study, a negative screen must not be used to give false reassurance, as these women may still be at increased risk. For example, if a first-degree relative has a significant thrombotic history but a negative thrombophilia screen, testing cannot offer any reassurance. Women found to have antithrombin deficiency or combined defects have the greatest risk. If a decision to use HRT is made, limited evidence suggests that the transdermal route might be safer. The comments made above regarding raloxifene, progestogens and tibolone are relevant here.

Women with a personal history of thrombosis on long-term warfarin

Hormone replacement therapy, raloxifene, progestogens and tibolone can be prescribed in these women, as the risk of recurrence should be very small provided anticoagulation continues.

Hormone replacement therapy and surgery
If HRT is stopped, the increased risk of VTE disappears rapidly, so HRT could be stopped 4 weeks before elective surgery. A more practical alternative is to continue HRT and ensure that adequate prophylaxis is given against VTE.

Obesity

Obesity is not a contraindication to HRT. However, as obesity increases the risk of VTE, transdermal delivery of oestrogen may be preferred.

Metabolic syndrome

The prime emphasis in management of the metabolic syndrome is to reduce underlying modifiable risk factors (obesity, physical inactivity and atherogenic diet) through lifestyle changes. There are specific recommendations for diet, exercise and weight loss of initially 7–10% of baseline weight in the first year with continued weight loss thereafter in order ultimately to achieve desirable weight (BMI <25 kg/m^2). If blood pressure, lipid and glycaemic control are not achieved through these interventions, pharmacological therapy is required. Again, the metabolic syndrome is not a contraindication to HRT, but the type and route of administration may need to be adjusted to take into account glycaemic and lipid control.

Endocrine disease
Diabetes mellitus

The number of people with diabetes is increasing due to population growth, ageing, urbanization, and increasing prevalence of obesity and physical inactivity. The prevalence of diabetes for all age groups worldwide was estimated to be 2.8% in 2000 and will increase to 4.4% in 2030. The total number of people with diabetes is projected to rise from 171 million in 2000 to 366 million in 2030. The prevalence of diabetes is higher in men than women, but there are more women with diabetes than men. Hormone replacement therapy seems to decrease the incidence of type 2 diabetes mellitus, as well as improving glycaemic control, with results varying according to the type and route of administration. It also improves lipid profiles, and transdermal delivery seems to decrease triglyceride levels in particular. While HRT may be beneficial in young, postmenopausal, diabetic women, especially those with premature ovarian failure, it cannot be advised for women older than 60 years with, or at high risk of, cardiovascular disease.

Cardioprotective adjunctive treatments (such as statins or low-dose aspirin) may be advised in diabetic women with risk factors for CHD and can be prescribed concomitantly with HRT. However, HRT is currently not recommended solely to prevent cardiovascular disease. Osteoporosis is reported as a potential complication of type 1 diabetes mellitus. In type 2 diabetes mellitus, the risk of hip fracture is higher than that in normoglycaemic women, despite higher bone mineral density (BMD). As types 1 and 2 diabetes increase the risk of endometrial cancer, women with these conditions must receive a progestogen if the uterus is intact.

Thyroid disease

Thyroid dysfunction is common in the general population, especially among older women. Serum thyroid autoantibodies, directed against thyroid peroxidase (TPO) and/or thyroglobulin (Tg), are detectable in up to 25% of women over age 60. Autoimmune hypothyroidism (with positive TPO and/or Tg antibodies) is 8–9 times more common in women than in men, and tends to become increasingly prevalent with age. Hypothyroidism is common, affecting 12–20% women over the age of 60. Hyperthyroidism is far less prevalent than hypothyroidism, affecting 2–4% women. In postmenopausal women, but not premenopausal women, overt thyrotoxicosis is associated with increased bone resorption, low BMD, and possibly fractures. Cortical bone is affected more severely than trabecular bone. Whether subclinical hyperthyroidism causes low BMD and/or increases fracture rates in postmenopausal women is controversial. Patients who present with hyperthyroidism should be screened for osteoporosis. Thyroid replacement is not a contraindication for HRT, but the dose of thyroxine may need to be increased because oestrogen can increase concentrations of thyroxine-binding globulin. Conversely, the dose of thyroid replacement may need to be reduced when HRT is stopped.

Neurological disease

Migraine

This condition is more common in women than men and is usually a condition of the reproductive years, starting during the teens and 20s. It is unusual for migraines to start after the age of 50 years. Menstruation is often a significant trigger, and the menopause marks a time of increased migraine. Hormone replacement therapy can help – not only by stabilizing fluctuations in oestrogen that are associated with migraine but also by relieving night sweats that disturb sleep. No good evidence supports the idea that HRT aggravates migraine. As migraine can be triggered by fluctuating concentrations of oestrogen, the transdermal route is favoured over the oral route, because it produces more stable levels of oestrogen. Too high an oestrogen dose can trigger migraine aura, which usually resolves as the dose is reduced. Unlike the contraceptive pill, no data suggest that the risk of ischaemic stroke is increased in women with migraine with aura who take HRT. Sequential progestogen treatment may be a trigger for migraine. The strategies that can be used are changing the type of progestogen, changing to continuous combined therapy and delivering the progestogen transdermally or into the uterus with the levonorgestrel device (see Chapter 6). Hormone replacement therapy can be taken concurrently with preventive or acute treatments such as triptans for migraine.

Epilepsy

Data about the menopause, HRT and epilepsy are limited. The incidence of epilepsy is higher in people over age 65 years than in younger adults. It is 90 per 100,000 among people aged 65–70 years, and increases to 150 per 100,000 in those older than 80 years. Cerebrovascular disease and neurodegenerative conditions such as Alzheimer's disease account for the increased incidence of new-onset epilepsy in the elderly. Severe epilepsy, with frequent seizures, advances the age of menopause by about 3–4 years. Seizure frequency may increase in the perimenopause, and this may be due to fluctuating ovarian steroid levels or sleep deprivation due to night sweats.

The type and dose of HRT have not been examined systematically. Limited data show worsening seizure frequency in oral HRT users. Of concern is that some antiepileptics are inducers of liver enzymes, and herbal preparations used for menopausal symptoms may interact with them (see Chapter 11). No data as yet confirm that the transdermal route is preferable to the oral route. Whether or not women who take oral therapy should take an increased dose (extrapolating from combined oral contraceptive usage) is not yet known.

Antiepileptic drug use promotes bone loss and increases the risk of osteo-porotic fracture. The problem is further compounded by the fact that seizures increase the risk of falls, especially in women with poorly controlled seizures. The exact mechanisms by which antiepileptic drugs promote bone loss leading to osteoporosis have not been completely elucidated. They are probably multifactorial and include hepatic microsomal enzyme induction leading to increased vitamin D catabolism, altered calcium absorption, secondary hyperparathyroidism, and a possible direct cytotoxic effect on bone cells. Data for bone thinning and frank osteoporosis are most robust for enzyme-inducing drugs such as phenytoin, phenobarbital, primidone, carba-mazepine and valproate. Less is known about the newer antiepileptic drugs such as topiramate, lamotrigine and levetiracetam. Recommendations have been made for women taking antiepileptic drugs at risk of osteoporosis. These include calcium and vitamin D supplementation. Women with epilepsy should be encouraged to exercise on a regular basis. Whether or not this supplemental strategy is effective in the face of strong, enzyme-inducing drugs is uncertain. Bone mineral density scans (dual energy X-ray absorptiometry scans) can help in identifying women at risk, although there are no currently agreed upon recommendations about their frequency in this group. Bisphosphonates should be considered in patients with known osteoporosis, although there are concerns about their long-term use (see Chapter 9).

Parkinson's disease

Oestrogen may protect against Parkinson's disease (PD). The risk of PD is greater in women with fewer years of fertility and earlier menopause. Premenopausal oophorectomy also increases the risk of parkinsonism compared to controls. This risk increases with younger age at oophorectomy.

Oestrogen may improve the symptoms of PD. It would seem, therefore, that HRT is not contraindicated and can be used in women taking drugs for PD. However, it is not known whether any particular regimen or route of administration is preferred. Nor is it known whether or not HRT can be used in women receiving deep brain stimulation.

Urinary problems

Urinary problems are common in postmenopausal women (see Chapter 3). Vaginal, but not oral, oestrogens, reduce the number of urinary tract infections in postmenopausal women, but the data are limited. Systemic oestrogens and raloxifene are ineffective in women with urinary incontinence but are not contraindicated in women taking drugs for either stress incontinence (eg duloxetine) or overactive bladder (eg oxybutinin, tolterodine, trospium hydrochloride, solfenacin). Vaginal oestrogen may help with symptoms of urgency.

Gastrointestinal conditions

Gallbladder disease

In the UK, about 8% of the population older than 40 years has gallstones; this figure increases to more than 20% in people older than 60 years. Randomized trials (HERS and WHI) have shown an increased risk of gallbladder disease with oral HRT (see Chapter 7). While the risk of gallbladder disease is less with transdermal oestrogen, it is not well established whether or not this route is better in women with pre-existing disease.

Liver disease

A non-oral route of oestrogen treatment is advised in women with liver disease to avoid the first liver pass, but the evidence is limited. Some types of liver disease, such as primary biliary cirrhosis, are associated with osteoporosis.

Inflammatory bowel disease

A major consideration in women with inflammatory bowel disease is the increased risk of osteoporosis, which may result from the disease itself or the long-term use of corticosteroids. The transdermal route of HRT is usually preferred to ensure adequate absorption in disease affecting the small bowel such as Crohn's disease.

Connective tissue disease

Rheumatoid arthritis

This is a systemic disorder that manifests itself primarily as a chronic, inflammatory polyarthropathy. It is six times more common in the sixth decade than in the second decade, and women are affected about 2.5 times more frequently than men. Women with rheumatoid arthritis are at increased risk of osteoporosis, and this may be related to disease severity, steroid use and immobility caused by the disease. Furthermore, bone resorption is increased in women with rheumatoid arthritis, and this is related to disease activity. The use of oestrogen- or non-oestrogen-based treatments will depend on the woman's symptoms, BMD and preference. No evidence shows that the use of HRT affects the risk of developing rheumatoid arthritis, and it does not induce flares in postmenopausal women.

Systemic lupus erythematosus

Systemic lupus erythematosus (SLE) is a rare multi-system rheumatic disease characterized by fever, arthritis, pleuropericarditis, skin rashes, grand mal seizures, kidney failure or pancytopaenia. It characteristically flares during pregnancy. The increased life expectancy of patients with SLE means that early cardiovascular mortality and glucocorticoid-associated bone loss are now important issues. Women with SLE are more likely to have premature menopause, osteoporosis and cardiovascular disease. Hormone replacement therapy can induce SLE flares and cardiovascular or venous thromboembolic events. Thus, it should not be used in women with active disease or those with antiphospholipid (aPL) antibodies. In general, it should only be used in patients without active disease, history of thrombosis or aPL antibodies. Non-oral oestrogen administration is recommended because of its lesser effect on coagulation. With regard to the progestogen, progesterone or pregnane derivatives are preferred because of their lesser effect on thrombotic risk. Otherwise, non-oestrogen-based strategies should be employed.

Other disorders

Respiratory problems

In women who have used systemic steroids, BMD needs to be assessed (see Chapter 5). There seems to be a small increase in the risk of asthma and asthma-like symptoms in women who use HRT. Its use, however, does not seem to worsen pre-existing asthma. No evidence exists with regard to tibolone or raloxifene.

Otosclerosis

This condition is inherited as a Mendelian dominant characteristic and leads to progressive deafness. Evidence suggests that pregnancy can aggravate this condition, and it can rarely worsen with oral contraceptives. No data, however, show that HRT causes deterioration of the disease. As the natural course of the disease is progressive, it is likely that hearing will become more impaired in women who use HRT in the long term.

After transplantation

Bone mass is reduced in a high percentage of patients after organ or marrow transplantation, with the prevalence of osteopenia or osteoporosis reported to be as high as 80%. Up to 65% of transplant recipients experience osteoporosis-related fracture, and the likelihood of developing such a serious outcome is dependent on pre-existing disease and immunosuppressive therapy. Post-transplant glucocorticoid therapy is thought to play a major role in the further reduction in bone mass seen in these patients. The additional role of other immunosuppressant treatments in bone loss is less clear, but some evidence suggests that cyclosporin A and tacrolimus (FK506) produce osteopenia as a result of high bone turnover. Anti-osteoporotic strategies need to be considered.

Renal failure

Patients with end-stage renal disease (ESRD) are at increased risk of early menopause, osteoporosis, cognitive dysfunction and cardiovascular disease. Data are needed in this population to define the benefits of oestrogen- and non-oestrogen-based treatments.

Further reading

Pelvic disorders

Fedele L, Bianchi S, Raffaelli R, Zanconato G. A randomized study of the effects of tibolone and transdermal oestrogen replacement therapy in postmenopausal women with uterine myomas. *Eur J Obstet Gynecol Reprod Biol* 2000;**88**:91–4.

Matorras R, Elorriaga MA, Pijoan JI, *et al.* Recurrence of endometriosis in women with bilateral adnexectomy (with or without total hysterectomy) who received hormone replacement therapy. *Fertil Steril* 2002;**77**:303–8.

Melton LJ 3rd, Leibson CL, Good AE, *et al.* Long-term fracture risk among women with proven endometriosis. *Fertil Steril* 2006;**86**:1576–83.

Sagsveen M, Farmer JE, Prentice A, Breeze A. Gonadotrophin-releasing hormone analogues for endometriosis: bone mineral density. *Cochrane Database Syst Rev* 2003;**4**:CD001297.

Soliman NF, Evans AJ. Malignancy arising in residual endometriosis following hysterectomy and hormone replacement therapy. *J Br Menopause Soc* 2004;**10**: 123–4.

Stratton P, Sinaii N, Segars J, *et al.* Return of chronic pelvic pain from endometriosis after raloxifene treatment: a randomized controlled trial. *Obstet Gynecol* 2008;**111**: 88–96.

Surrey ES, Hornstein MD. Prolonged GnRH agonist and add-back therapy for symptomatic endometriosis: long-term follow-up. *Obstet Gynecol* 2002;**99**:709–19.

Wu T, Chen X, Xie L. Selective estrogen receptor modulators (SERMs) for uterine leiomyomas. *Cochrane Database Syst Rev* 2007;**4**:CD005287.

Yang CH, Lee JN, Hsu SC, *et al.* Effect of hormone replacement therapy on uterine fibroids in postmenopausal women – a 3-year study. *Maturitas* 2002;**43**:35–9.

Zupi E, Marconi D, Sbracia M, *et al.* Add-back therapy in the treatment of endometriosis-associated pain. *Fertil Steril* 2004;**82**:1303–8.

Cardiovascular disease

Barrett-Connor E, Mosca L, Collins P, *et al.*; Raloxifene Use for The Heart (RUTH) Trial Investigators. Effects of raloxifene on cardiovascular events and breast cancer in postmenopausal women. *N Engl J Med* 2006;**355**:125–37.

Cagnacci A, Baldassari F, Arangino S, *et al.* Administration of tibolone decreases 24 h heart rate but not blood pressure of post-menopausal women. *Maturitas* 2004;**48**: 155–60.

Canonico M, Oger E, Plu-Bureau G, *et al.*; Estrogen and Thromboembolism Risk (ESTHER) Study Group. Hormone therapy and venous thromboembolism among postmenopausal women: impact of the route of estrogen administration and progestogens: the ESTHER study. *Circulation* 2007;**115**:840–5.

Canonico M, Plu-Bureau G, Lowe GD, Scarabin PY. Hormone replacement therapy and risk of venous thromboembolism in postmenopausal women: systematic review and meta-analysis. *BMJ* 2008;**336**:1227–31.

Curb JD, Prentice RL, Bray PF, *et al.* Venous thrombosis and conjugated equine estrogen in women without a uterus. *Arch Intern Med* 2006;**166**:772–80.

Cushman M, Kuller LH, Prentice R, *et al.* Estrogen plus progestin and risk of venous thrombosis. *JAMA* 2004;**292**:1573–80.

de Valk-de Roo GW, Stehouwer CD, Meijer P, *et al.* Both raloxifene and estrogen reduce major cardiovascular risk factors in healthy postmenopausal women: a 2-year, placebo-controlled study. *Arterioscler Thromb Vasc Biol* 1999;**19**:2993–3000.

Grady D, Wenger NK, Herrington D, *et al.* Postmenopausal hormone therapy increases risk for venous thromboembolic disease. The Heart and Estrogen/progestin Replacement Study. *Ann Intern Med* 2000;**132**:689–96.

Herrington DM, Vittinghoff E, Howard TD, *et al.* Factor V Leiden, hormone replacement therapy, and risk of venous thromboembolic events in women with coronary disease. *Arterioscler Thromb Vasc Biol* 2002;**22**:1012–17.

Ichikawa J, Sumino H, Ichikawa S, Ozaki M. Different effects of transdermal and oral hormone replacement therapy on the renin-angiotensin system, plasma bradykinin level, and blood pressure of normotensive postmenopausal women. *Am J Hypertens* 2006;**19**:744–9.

Kaaja RJ. Metabolic syndrome and the menopause. *Menopause Int* 2008;**14**:21–5.

Keeling DM. Hormone replacement therapy, thrombosis and thrombophilia. *J Br Menopause Soc* 2005;**11**:74–5.

Mueck AO, Seeger H. Effect of hormone therapy on BP in normotensive and hypertensive postmenopausal women. *Maturitas* 2004;**49**:189–203.

Prendergast BD, Harrison JL, Naber CK. Commentary on endocarditis prophylaxis: a quaint custom or medical necessity? *Heart* 2008;**94**:931–4.

Royal College of Obstetricians and Gynaecologists. *Hormone Replacement Therapy and Venous Thromboembolism*. Guideline 19. London: Royal College of Obstetricians and Gynaecologists, 2004.

Steiner AZ, Hodis HN, Lobo RA, *et al.* Postmenopausal oral estrogen therapy and blood pressure in normotensive and hypertensive subjects: the Estrogen in the Prevention of Atherosclerosis Trial. *Menopause* 2005;**12**:728–33.

Stevenson JC. Metabolic effects of hormone replacement therapy. *J Br Menopause Soc* 2004;**10**:157–61.

Endocrine disease

Ahmed LA, Joakimsen RM, Berntsen GK, *et al.* Diabetes mellitus and the risk of non-vertebral fractures: the Tromsø study. *Osteoporos Int* 2006;**17**:495–500.

Anderson KE, Anderson E, Mink PJ, *et al.* Diabetes and endometrial cancer in the Iowa women's health study. *Cancer Epidemiol Biomarkers Prev* 2001;**10**:611–16.

Arafah BM. Increased need for thyroxine in women with hypothyroidism during estrogen therapy. *N Engl J Med* 2001;**344**:1743–9.

Auryan S, Itamar R. Gender-specific care of diabetes mellitus: particular considerations in the management of diabetic women. *Diabetes Obes Metab* 2008;**10**: 1135–56.

Bonds DE, Larson JC, Schwartz AV, *et al.* Risk of fracture in women with type 2 diabetes: the Women's Health Initiative Observational Study. *J Clin Endocrinol Metab* 2006;**91**:3404–10.

Canaris GJ, Manowitz NR, Mayor G, *et al.* The Colorado thyroid disease prevalence study. *Arch Intern Med* 2000;**160**:526–34.

Cummings SR, Nevitt MC, Browner WS, *et al.* Risk factors for hip fracture in white women. Study of Osteoporotic Fractures Research Group. *N Engl J Med* 1995;**332**: 767–73.

Ferrara A, Quesenberry CP, Karter AJ, *et al.* Current use of unopposed estrogen and estrogen plus progestin and the risk of acute myocardial infarction among women with diabetes: the Northern California Kaiser Permanente Diabetes Registry, 1995–1998. *Circulation* 2003;**107**:43–8.

Hollowell J, Staehling NW, Flanders WD, *et al.* Serum TSH, T(4), and thyroid antibodies in the United States population (1988 to 1994): National Health and Nutrition Examination Survey (NHANES III). *J Clin Endocrinol Metab* 2002;**87**: 489–99.

Kanaya A, Herrington D, Vittinghoff E, *et al.* Glycemic effects of postmenopausal hormone therapy: the Heart and Estrogen/progestin Replacement Study. *Ann Intern Med* 2003;**138**:1–9.

Khoo CL, Perera M. Diabetes and the menopause. *J Br Menopause Soc* 2005;**11**:6–11.

Margolis KL, Bonds DE, Rodabough RJ, *et al.* Effect of oestrogen plus progestin on the incidence of diabetes in postmenopausal women: results from the Women's Health Initiative Hormone Trial. *Diabetologia* 2004;**47**:1175–87.

Pearce EN. Thyroid dysfunction in perimenopausal and postmenopausal women. *Menopause Int* 2007;**13**:8–13

Rossi R, Origliani G, Modena M. Transdermal 17β estradiol and risk of developing type 2 diabetes in a population of healthy, nonobese postmenopausal women. *Diabetes Care* 2004;**27**:645–9.

Sawin CT, Castelli WP, Hershman JM, *et al.* The aging thyroid: thyroid deficiency in the Framingham Study. *Arch Intern Med* 1985;**145**:1386–8.

Schwartz A, Sellmeyer D, Ensrud K, *et al.* Older women with diabetes have an increased risk of fracture: a prospective study. *J Clin Endocrinol Metab* 2001;**86**: 32–8.

Wild S, Roglic G, Green A, *et al.* Global prevalence of diabetes: estimates for the year 2000 and projections for 2030. *Diabetes Care* 2004;**27**:1047–53.

Zendehdel K, Nyren O, Ostenson CG, *et al.* Cancer incidence in patients with type 1 diabetes mellitus: a population-based cohort study in Sweden. *J Natl Cancer Inst* 2003;**95**:1797–800.

Neurological disease

Abbasi F, Krumholz A, Kittner SJ, Langenberg P. Effects of menopause on seizures in women with epilepsy. *Epilepsia* 1999;**40**:205–10.

Brandes JL. The influence of estrogen on migraine: a systematic review. *JAMA* 2006;**295**:1824–30.

Currie LJ, Harrison MB, Trugman JM, et al. Postmenopausal estrogen use affects risk for Parkinson disease. *Arch Neurol* 2004;**61**:886–8.

Ensrud KE, Walczak TS, Blackwell T, et al. Antiepileptic drug use increases rates of bone loss in older women: a prospective study. *Neurology* 2004;**62**:2051–7.

Green PS, Simpkins JW. Neuroprotective effects of estrogens: potential mechanisms of action. *Int J Dev Neurosci* 2000;**18**:347–58.

Harden CL, Pulver MC, Ravdin L, Jacobs AR. The effect of menopause and peri-menopause on the course of epilepsy. *Epilepsia* 1999;**40**:1402–7.

Harden CL, Koppel BS, Herzog AG, et al. Seizure frequency is associated with age of menopause in women with epilepsy. *Neurology* 2003;**61**:451–5.

Harden CL, Herzog AG, Nikolov BG, et al. Hormone replacement therapy in women with epilepsy: a randomized, double-blind, placebo-controlled study. *Epilepsia* 2006;**47**:1447–51.

Koppel BS, Harden CL, Nikolov BG, Labar DR. An analysis of lifetime fractures in women with epilepsy. *Acta Neurol Scand* 2005;**111**:225–8.

Loder E, Rizzoli P, Golub J. Hormonal management of migraine associated with menses and the menopause: a clinical review. *Headache* 2007;**47**:329–40.

MacGregor EA. Menstrual migraine. In: Rees M, Hope S, Ravnikar V, eds. *The Abnormal Menstrual Cycle*. Abingdon: Taylor and Francis, 2005:197–218.

MacGregor EA. Migraine, the menopause and hormone replacement therapy: a clinical review. *J Fam Plann Reprod Health Care* 2007;**33**:245–9.

Pack AM, Morrell MJ. Epilepsy and bone health in adults. *Epilepsy Behav* 2004;**5**(Suppl 2):S24–9.

Price MD, Shulman LM. Management of Parkinson's disease in older women. *Menopause Int* 2008;**14**:38–9.

Ragonese P, D'Amelio M, Salemi G, et al. Risk of Parkinson disease in women: effect of reproductive characteristics. *Neurology* 2004;**62**:2010–14.

Rocca WA, Bower JH, Maraganore DM, et al. Increased risk of parkinsonism in women who underwent oophorectomy before menopause. *Neurology* 2008;**70**:200–9.

Sethi NK, Harden CL. Epilepsy in older women. *Menopause Int* 2008;**14**;85–7.

Sheth RD, Wesolowski CA, Jacob JC, et al. Effect of carbamazepine and valproate on bone mineral density. *J Pediatr* 1995;**127**:256–62.

Tsang KL, Ho SL, Lo SK. Estrogen improves motor disability in parkinsonian post-menopausal women with motor fluctuations. *Neurology* 2000;**54**:2292–8.

Urinary problems

Hendrix SL, Cochrane BB, Nygaard IE, et al. Effects of estrogen with and without progestin on urinary incontinence. *JAMA* 2005;**293**:935–48.

Perrotta C, Aznar M, Mejia R, *et al*. Oestrogens for preventing recurrent urinary tract infection in postmenopausal women. *Cochrane Database Syst Rev* 2008;2: CD005131.

Simunić V, Banović I, Ciglar S, *et al*. Local estrogen treatment in patients with urogenital symptoms. *Int J Gynaecol Obstet* 2003;**82**:187–97.

Steinauer JE, Waetjen LE, Vittinghoff E, *et al*. Postmenopausal hormone therapy: does it cause incontinence? *Obstet Gynecol* 2005;**106**:940–5.

Waetjen LE, Brown JS, Modelska K, *et al*.; MORE Study Group. Effect of raloxifene on urinary incontinence: a randomized controlled trial. *Obstet Gynecol* 2004;**103**: 261–6.

Waetjen LE, Brown JS, Vittinghoff E, *et al*. The effect of ultralow-dose transdermal estradiol on urinary incontinence in postmenopausal women. *Obstet Gynecol* 2005;**106**:946–52.

Gastrointestinal conditions

Cirillo DJ, Wallace RB, Rodabough RJ, *et al*. Effect of estrogen therapy on gallbladder disease. *JAMA* 2005;**293**:330–9.

Hulley S, Grady D, Bush T, *et al*. Randomized trial of estrogen plus progestin for secondary prevention of coronary heart disease in postmenopausal women. Heart and Estrogen/progestin Replacement Study (HERS) Research Group. *JAMA* 1998;**280**:605–13.

Johnson CD. ABC of the upper gastrointestinal tract: upper abdominal pain: gall bladder. *BMJ* 2001;**323**:1170–3.

Ormarsdottir S, Mallmin H, Naessen T, *et al*. An open, randomized, controlled study of transdermal hormone replacement therapy on the rate of bone loss in primary biliary cirrhosis. *J Intern Med* 2004;**256**:63–9.

Tilg H, Moschen AR, Kaser A, *et al*. Gut, inflammation and osteoporosis: basic and clinical concepts. *Gut* 2008;**57**:684–94.

Connective tissue disease

Bernatsky S, Boivin JF, Joseph L, *et al*. Mortality in systemic lupus erythematosus. *Arthritis Rheum* 2006;**54**:2550–7.

Buyon JP, Petri MA, Kim MY, *et al*. The effect of combined estrogen and progesterone hormone replacement therapy on disease activity in systemic lupus erythematosus: a randomized trial. *Ann Intern Med* 2005;**142**:953–62.

Canonico M, Oger E, Plu-Bureau G, *et al*.; Estrogen and Thromboembolism Risk (ESTHER) Study Group. Hormone therapy and venous thromboembolism among postmenopausal women: impact of the route of estrogen administration and progestogens: the ESTHER study. *Circulation* 2007;**115**:840–5.

D'Elia HF, Larsen A, Mattsson LA, *et al*. Influence of hormone replacement therapy on disease progression and bone mineral density in rheumatoid arthritis. *J Rheumatol* 2003;**30**:1456–63.

Gompel A, Piette JC. Systemic lupus erythematosus and hormone replacement therapy. *Menopause Int* 2007;**13**:65–70.

Lange U, Illgner U, Teichmann J, Schleenbecker H. Skeletal benefit after one year of risedronate therapy in patients with rheumatoid arthritis and glucocorticoid-induced osteoporosis: a prospective study. *Int J Clin Pharmacol Res* 2004;**24**:33–8.

Lee C, Ramsey-Goldman R. Osteoporosis in systemic lupus erythematosus mechanisms. *Rheum Dis Clin North Am* 2005;**31**:363–85.

Lems WF, Lodder MC, Lips P, *et al.* Positive effect of alendronate on bone mineral density and markers of bone turnover in patients with rheumatoid arthritis on chronic treatment with low-dose prednisone: a randomized, double-blind, placebo-controlled trial. *Osteoporos Int* 2006;**17**:716–23.

Lodder MC, de Jong Z, Kostense PJ, *et al.* Bone mineral density in patients with rheumatoid arthritis: relation between disease severity and low bone mineral density. *Ann Rheum Dis* 2004;**63**:1576–80.

Yee CS, Crabtree N, Skan J, *et al.* Prevalence and predictors of fragility fractures in systemic lupus erythematosus. *Ann Rheum Dis* 2005;**64**:111–13.

Other disorders

Barr RG, Wentowski CC, Grodstein F, *et al.* Prospective study of postmenopausal hormone use and newly diagnosed asthma and chronic obstructive pulmonary disease. *Arch Intern Med* 2004;**164**:379–86.

Dolgos S, Hartmann A, Bønsnes S, *et al.* Determinants of bone mass in end-stage renal failure patients at the time of kidney transplantation. *Clin Transplant* 2008;**22**:462–8.

Kramer HM, Curhan GC, Singh A. Permanent cessation of menses and post-menopausal hormone use in dialysis-dependent women: the HELP study. *Am J Kidney Dis* 2003;**41**:643–50.

Ramsey-Goldman R, Dunn JE, Dunlop DD, *et al.* Increased risk of fracture in patients receiving solid organ transplants. *J Bone Miner Res* 1999;**14**:456–63.

Shane E, Addesso V, Namerow PB, *et al.* Alendronate versus calcitriol for the prevention of bone loss after cardiac transplantation. *N Engl J Med* 2004;**350**:767–76.

Stein E, Ebeling P, Shane E. Post-transplantation osteoporosis. *Endocrinol Metab Clin North Am* 2007;**36**:937–63, viii.

Thompson W. Otosclerosis and hormone replacement therapy: fact or fiction? *J Br Menopause Soc* 1999;**5**:54.

14 Women at increased risk of developing cancer or with a previous malignancy

> **Breast cancer**
> **Gynaecological cancer**
> **Other cancers**
> **Further reading**

Women with previous cancer or at increased risk of developing a malignancy may be wary of taking oestrogen. Most cancers are not hormone dependent and thus oestrogen replacement is not contraindicated. The areas of controversy arise in breast, gynaecological and colorectal cancers, and malignant melanoma.

Breast cancer

Women may be placed at increased risk of breast cancer by family history or high-risk benign breast condition.

Family history of breast cancer

Little evidence shows that the use of hormone replacement therapy (HRT) in patients with family history of breast cancer will further increase their risk, but, for the most part, studies have failed to document family history accurately. Furthermore among postmenopausal women with a BRCA1 mutation, HRT use is not associated with an increased risk of breast cancer. No evidence supports the safety of herbal medicines in these women. Any woman with a significant family history should be referred to a specialist breast clinic to determine her personal risk, without which informed decisions cannot be made (see Chapter 5).

Benign breast disease

The most widely recognized and accepted classification of benign breast conditions is histological and categorizes benign changes according to the subsequent risk of cancer development. Most benign conditions are not associated with a significant increase in risk; therefore, in clinical practice, once a histological diagnosis is confirmed, regular follow-up or surveillance is not indicated for most women. Epithelial atypia (ie ductal or lobular atypical hyperplasia) is associated with a four- to fivefold increase in risk, but the optimal surveillance (including duration) and other prevention strategies for women with biopsy-proven atypia are unknown. Although HRT may be associated with mastalgia and promotion of breast cysts, no convincing evidence shows that the risk of breast cancer is increased in patients with benign disease. Failure to categorize benign disease accurately, however, prevents determination of whether or not women involved in these studies were at significantly increased risk of breast cancer.

Overall, there is no evidence that use of HRT (unopposed or combined) has an additive impact on risk, studies suggesting that HRT entails a similar degree of risk to that in women who are at average (ie population) risk. The most important factor contributing to increased risk in these groups of women is their baseline breast cancer risk, which is determined by their family history or personal history of benign breast change. Therefore, it follows that, for example, if a woman's baseline risk is increased fourfold by specific family history or high-risk benign breast condition, use of HRT is associated with a greater absolute risk than that entailed by use if at baseline population risk.

Previous breast cancer

Survivors of breast cancer with menopausal symptoms pose a management problem, as conventional advice is to avoid the use of exogenous oestrogens. Survival rates for breast cancer have been improving for more than 20 years. The estimated relative 5-year survival rate for women diagnosed in England and Wales in 2001–3 was 80%, compared with only 52% for women diagnosed in 1971–5 (Figure 14.1). The estimated relative 20-year survival rate for women with breast cancer has gone from 44% in the early 1990s to 64% for the most recent period. This means that management of breast cancer survivors is an important problem. The issues are not only menopausal symptoms but also increased risk of osteoporotic fracture and cardiovascular disease as well as a second cancer.

Most observational studies of patients with breast cancer who have been prescribed systemic HRT have not shown an adverse effect on survival; however, these involved small numbers of patients, with short-term follow-up, and as they were uncontrolled, the results are open to bias. Preliminary analysis of two randomized trials in Scandinavia (HABITS and Stockholm studies) has shown contradictory results. The HABITS study reported increased recurrence risk, whereas in the Stockholm study recurrence was not increased. In the latter study, more women used concomitant tamoxifen

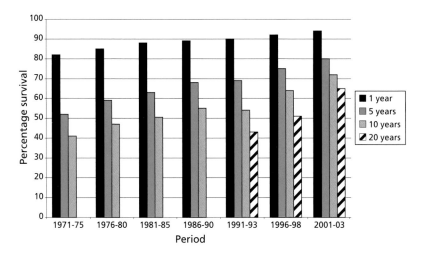

Figure 14.1 Age-standardized relative survival (%) at 1, 5, 10 and 20 years since diagnosis, female breast cancer, England and Wales, 1971–2003. Adapted with permission from info.cancerresearchuk.org/cancerstats/types/breast/survival

and had long-cycle combined HRT. The adverse results of the HABITS study, although based on a very small number of clinical events, resulted in the premature cessation of the Stockholm study (in which no increase in risk was found). It also halted the National UK randomized trial of HRT in symptomatic women with early-stage breast cancer. Currently, the effect of HRT is uncertain, and it is important to appreciate problems that arise from over-interpretation of preliminary outcomes – whatever effect is shown. The randomized LIBERATE trial of tibolone in survivors of breast cancer was discontinued in 2007 due to an increase in the risk of recurrence.

Management of menopausal symptoms
Hot flushes and night sweats occur in about two-thirds of women with breast cancer and often are a consequence of their treatment. Most cancers are hormone sensitive and women have therapy designed to reduce oestrogen synthesis or antagonize its effects (eg ovarian suppression following chemotherapy, medical castration with luteinizing hormone-releasing hormone analogues, aromatase inhibitors, tamoxifen). Iatrogenic symptoms appear to be more severe and longer-lasting than symptoms arising from natural menopause. In addition to vasomotor symptoms, breast cancer therapy is associated with increased urogenital symptoms (vaginal dryness, dyspareunia), fatigue, mood disturbance and joint pain.

Systemic oestrogen-based HRT is usually avoided, especially in women with oestrogen receptor-positive tumours. The pharmacological alternatives are clonidine, selective serotonin-reuptake inhibitors (paroxetine, fluoxetine and citalopram), serotonin-norepinephrine reuptake inhibitors (SNRIs) (venlafaxine), and gabapentin. However, efficacy has been found only in short- and not long-term studies (up to 12 weeks). Desvenlafaxine (an SNRI) is currently being evaluated for the treatment of hot flushes in breast cancer survivors. Progestogens such as megestrol acetate may be helpful, but in effective doses they can cause weight gain, and there are concerns about safety, as the Women's Health Initiative study found an increased risk of breast cancer in combined HRT users.

The safety and efficacy of alternative and complementary therapies are unknown. Some herbal preparations may contain oestrogenic compounds; therefore, caution should be exercised in women with hormone-responsive disease.

For urogenital symptoms, water-based lubricants and bioadhesive moisturizers may help. However, low-dose vaginal oestradiol and oestriol, used in the recommended doses, are not contraindicated. Fatigue appears to affect about 20% of patients and persists for many years. There are no well-established management strategies, but yoga may be helpful.

Conserving the skeleton

Chemotherapy-induced ovarian failure increases the risk of osteoporosis and vertebral fracture. Tamoxifen, as an adjuvant therapy for breast cancer, increases spine and hip bone mineral density (BMD) in postmenopausal but not premenopausal patients. No significant reduction in osteoporotic fractures in the former group of women has yet been reported, however, and the use of tamoxifen does not appear to reverse the deleterious impact of chemotherapy on bone density.

However, other adjuvant regimens, such as gonadotrophin-releasing hormone analogues or aromatase inhibitors (anastrazole and letrozole), increase bone loss and induce osteoporosis, increasing the risk of fracture. Some experts recommend that all women starting aromatase inhibitor therapy should be assessed for risk of osteoporosis and have their BMD measured. Therefore, it is advised that breast cancer patients exercise regularly and take calcium (1500 mg) and vitamin D (800 IU/day) supplements. Patients with existing osteopenia and osteoporosis should be evaluated for conditions that further deteriorate skeletal health, such as hyperthyroidism. Bisphosphonates should be considered in osteoporotic women and probably be administered as long as aromatase inhibitor therapy is continued. Bisphosphonates may also reduce the risk of bone metastasis.

Cardiovascular disease

Congestive heart failure can occur after chemotherapy. This occurs in around 0.5–1.0% of women treated with standard anthracycline-based chemotherapy. Risk factors for cardiotoxicity include older age, pre-existing cardiac disease, higher cumulative dose of anthracycline, and radiation to the heart. The addition of trastuzumab may increase the risk of cardiac events.

Some, but not all, studies have found that radiotherapy after mastectomy also causes increased risk of cardiovascular morbidity and mortality. Tamoxifen is not associated with increased risk of coronary heart disease. Furthermore, fewer cardiovascular events have been found in tamoxifen than in letrozole users. However, tamoxifen is associated with two to three times increased risk of thromboembolic events.

Risk of a second cancer

While awareness is high of breast cancer recurrence many decades after the initial diagnosis, there is now increasing concern about the risk of developing unrelated cancer. A large cohort of women ($n = 525,527$) with primary breast cancer from 13 cancer registries in Europe, Canada, Australia and Singapore between 1943 and 2000 has provided useful information. Specific increased risk (SIR) was noted for stomach cancer (SIR = 1.35), colorectal cancer (SIR = 1.22), lung cancer (SIR = 1.24), soft tissue sarcoma (SIR = 2.25), melanoma (SIR = 1.29), non-melanoma (SIR = 1.58), endometrial cancer (SIR = 1.52), ovarian cancer (SIR = 1.48), kidney cancer (SIR = 1.27), thyroid cancer (SIR = 1.62) and leukaemia (SIR = 1.52). The increased risk of endometrial cancer with tamoxifen is well known. Routine screening is not recommended; however, tamoxifen users with vaginal bleeding should be urgently referred for endometrial assessment.

Fertility and contraception

The fact that young women are surviving breast cancer means that fertility and contraception are important issues. The percentage of patients who have full-term pregnancies after breast cancer diagnosis is very small, and there may be an increased chance of spontaneous abortion (25%) or pregnancy complications. Pregnancy after breast cancer does not appear to affect survival adversely. There has been debate about how long women should wait before trying to conceive. Current medical advice given to premenopausal women with a diagnosis of breast cancer is to wait 2 years before attempting to conceive. However, in women with localized disease, early conception, 6 months after completing their treatment, is unlikely to reduce survival.

What contraception to use is a controversial issue. The following recommendations of the Council of the Society of Obstetricians and

Gynaecologists of Canada and of the Society of Gynecologic Oncologists of Canada, published in 2006, are a useful guide:

- Non-hormonal contraceptive methods should be used as first-line options in the breast cancer survivor.
- Depot medroxyprogesterone acetate use in a breast cancer survivor can be considered in circumstances where contraceptive or non-contraceptive benefits outweigh any unknown potential increase in recurrence risk.
- Use of progestogen-only pills in a breast cancer survivor may be considered in a situation where known benefits outweigh any unknown potential increase in recurrence risk.
- Use of the levonorgestrel intrauterine system in the breast cancer survivor can be considered if the unique contraceptive or non-contraceptive benefits outweigh the risk of an unknown effect on recurrence.

Gynaecological cancer

Ovarian, cervical, vaginal and vulval cancers are not oestrogen-dependent conditions, and oestrogen replacement is not contraindicated. Endometrial carcinoma is often listed in data sheets as an absolute contraindication to HRT. Data for use of tibolone and raloxifene are scant. Non-hormonal therapies for osteoporosis or menopausal symptoms are not contraindicated. The safety of complementary and alternative medicines, such as botanicals, is unknown.

Ovarian cancer

Studies of oestrogen replacement do not show a detrimental effect on survival. They are mainly observational. There is a paucity of data regarding endometrioid ovarian cancer. Its potential oestrogen dependence intuitively suggests the use of combined oestrogen-progestogen HRT rather than oestrogen alone. The rationale of progestogen addition is to suppress any oestrogen-stimulated growth, but there is no strong scientific evidence to support this practice.

BRCA1 and BRCA2 mutation carriers

Mutations such as *BRCA1* and *BRCA2* increase the risk of ovarian cancer. The average cumulative lifetime risk has been estimated as up to 60% for *BRCA1* and up to 40% for *BRCA2* mutation carriers. Bilateral prophylactic oophorectomy is increasingly being performed in these women, leading to early ovarian failure. Data regarding HRT use in *BRCA* carriers are limited and show no adverse effect.

Endometrial cancer

No data show an increased risk of recurrence or mortality with HRT in women with a history of endometrial cancer. The few published studies have failed to demonstrate increase in recurrence or death rate among HRT users, and thus its use in endometrial cancer survivors does not seem to be contraindicated. The studies are limited by small sample size, retrospective design, selection bias, variation in hormone preparations and disease severity. Therefore, although the available data are encouraging, the question of whether or not HRT should be given after endometrial cancer remains unanswered. The American College of Obstetricians and Gynaecologists (ACOG) has stated that there is insufficient evidence to support specific recommendations of the use of HRT in women with a history of endometrial cancer. They have commented that, although the indications for use of HRT in this population are similar to those for other women, patients should be selected on the basis of prognostic indicators such as depth of invasion, grading and cell type, and the risk the patient is willing to take.

Cervical cancer

Cervical cancer is not an oestrogen-dependent disease, and thus HRT is not contraindicated. In women who have had hysterectomy, oestrogen only can be used. However, in those treated by chemoradiotherapy and in whom the uterus is retained, it cannot be assumed that all the endometrium has been destroyed. Indeed, there are reports of persisting functioning endometrial tissue and cancer after definitive radiation treatment for invasive cervical cancer. In women who retain their uterus, progestogen must be added to the oestrogen. Moreover, ovarian activity may return, and an effective form of contraception needs to be advised, since the outcomes of pregnancy in this situation are unknown. Cervical intraepithelial neoplasia (CIN) is also not a contraindication to oestrogen use.

Other cancers

Colorectal cancer

Women are less susceptible to colorectal cancer and benign colonic adenomas than men. Large-scale, randomized and observational studies show that HRT users have a reduced risk of colorectal cancer. However, there are no data in women at increased risk of the disease or with previous cancer.

Malignant melanoma

Malignant melanoma is a controversial area. It generally is accepted that no association exists between the risk of melanoma and the use of HRT. Reports of a relation between the prognosis of melanoma and HRT are contradictory. Oestrogen receptors are present on melanomas, but it seems unlikely that oestradiol has a direct effect on melanogenesis.

Lentigo maligna is the precursor of lentigo maligna melanoma. It is most common in the eighth decade, is found on the cheek or neck, and correlates closely with exposure to ultraviolet radiation. That lentigo maligna possesses both oestrogen and progesterone receptors suggests a possible role of these steroids in malignant transformation.

Further reading

Breast cancer

Bower JE, Woolery A, Sternlieb B, Garet D. Yoga for cancer patients and survivors. *Cancer Control* 2005;**12**:165–71.

Chen Z, Maricic M, Bassford TL, *et al.* Fracture risk among breast cancer survivors: results from the Women's Health Initiative Observational Study. *Arch Intern Med* 2005;**165**:552–8.

Dalberg K, Eriksson J, Holmberg L. Birth outcome in women with previously treated breast cancer – a population-based cohort study from Sweden. *PLoS Med* 2006;**3**: e336.

Dupont WD, Page DL, Parl FF, *et al.* Estrogen replacement therapy in women with a history of proliferative breast disease. *Cancer* 1999;**85**:1277–83.

Eisen A, Lubinski J, Gronwald J, *et al.*; Hereditary Breast Cancer Clinical Study Group. Hormone therapy and the risk of breast cancer in BRCA1 mutation carriers. *J Natl Cancer Inst* 2008;**100**:1361–7.

Glaus A, Boehme Ch, Thürlimann B, *et al.* Fatigue and menopausal symptoms in women with breast cancer undergoing hormonal cancer treatment. *Ann Oncol* 2006;**17**:801–6.

Hartmann LC, Sellers TA, Frost MH, *et al.* Benign breast disease and the risk of breast cancer. *N Engl J Med* 2005;**353**:229–37.

Holmberg L, Anderson H. HABITS (hormonal replacement therapy after breast cancer – is it safe?), a randomised comparison: trial stopped. *Lancet* 2004;**363**: 453–5.

Holmberg L, Iversen O-E, Rudenstam CM, *et al.*; HABITS Study Group. Increased risk of recurrence after hormone replacement therapy in breast cancer survivors. *J Natl Cancer Inst* 2008;**100**:475–82.

Ives A, Saunders C, Bulsara M, Semmens J. Pregnancy after breast cancer: population based study. *BMJ* 2007;**334**:194.

Livial Intervention Following Breast Cancer; Efficacy, Recurrence and Tolerability Endpoints (LIBERATE). clinicaltrials.gov/ct2/show/NCT00408863?intr=%22 Tibolone%22&rank=7.

McNaught J, Reid RL; SOGC/GOC Joint Ad Hoc Committee on Breast Cancer, Provencher DM, Lea RH, Jeffrey JF, *et al.* Progesterone-only and non-hormonal contraception in the breast cancer survivor: Joint Review and Committee Opinion of the Society of Obstetricians and Gynaecologists of Canada and the Society of Gynecologic Oncologists of Canada. *J Obstet Gynaecol Can* 2006;28:616–39.

Mellemkjaer L, Friis S, Olsen JH, *et al.* Risk of second cancer among women with breast cancer. *Int J Cancer* 2006;118:2285–92.

Mom CH, Buijs C, Willemse PH, *et al.* Hot flushes in breast cancer patients. *Crit Rev Oncol Hematol* 2006;57:63–77.

O'Meara ES, Rossing MA, Daling JR, *et al.* Hormone replacement therapy after a diagnosis of breast cancer in relation to recurrence and mortality. *J Natl Cancer Inst* 2001;93:754–61.

Rebbeck TR, Friebel T, Wagner T, *et al.*; PROSE Study Group. Effect of short-term hormone replacement therapy on breast cancer risk reduction after bilateral prophylactic oophorectomy in *BRCA1* and *BRCA2* mutation carriers: the PROSE Study Group. *J Clin Oncol* 2005;23:7804–10.

Reid DM, Doughty J, Eastell R, *et al.* Guidance for the management of breast cancer treatment-induced bone loss: a consensus position statement from a UK Expert Group. *Cancer Treat Rev* 2008;34(Suppl 1):S3–18.

Rohan TE, Miller AB. Hormone replacement therapy and risk of benign proliferative epithelial disorders of the breast. *Eur J Cancer Prev* 1999;8:123–30.

Rozenberg S, Antoine C, Carly B, *et al.* Improving quality of life after breast cancer: prevention of other diseases. *Menopause Int* 2007;13:71–4.

Santen RJ, Mansel R. Benign breast disorders. *N Engl J Med* 2005;353:275–85.

Speroff L, Gass M, Constantine G, Olivier S; Study 315 Investigators. Efficacy and tolerability of desvenlafaxine succinate treatment for menopausal vasomotor symptoms: a randomized controlled trial. *Obstet Gynecol* 2008;111:77–87.

von Schoultz E, Rutqvist LE. Menopausal hormone therapy after breast cancer: the Stockholm randomized trial. *J Natl Cancer Inst* 2005;97:533–5.

Gynaecological cancer

Antoniou A, Pharoah PD, Narod S, *et al.* Average risks of breast and ovarian cancer associated with *BRCA1* or *BRCA2* mutations detected in case series unselected for family history: a combined analysis of 22 studies. *Am J Hum Genet* 2003;72:1117–30.

Barakat RR, Bundy BN, Spirtos NM, *et al.*; Gynecologic Oncology Group Study. Randomized double-blind trial of estrogen replacement therapy versus placebo in stage I or II endometrial cancer: a Gynecologic Oncology Group Study. *J Clin Oncol* 2006;24:587–92.

Bebar S, Ursic-Vrscaj M. Hormone replacement therapy after epithelial ovarian cancer treatment. *Eur J Gynaecol Oncol* 2000;21:192–6.

Committee on Gynecologic Practice. ACOG committee opinion. Hormone replacement therapy in women treated for endometrial cancer. Number 234, May 2000 (replaces number 126, August 1993). *Int J Gynaecol Obstet* 2001;73:283–4.

Guidozzi F, Daponte A. Estrogen replacement therapy for ovarian carcinoma survivors: a randomized controlled trial. *Cancer* 1999;**86**:1013–18.

Habeshaw T, Pinion SB. The incidence of persistent functioning endometrial tissue following successful radiotherapy for cervical carcinoma. *Int J Gynecol Cancer* 1992;**2**:332–5.

Kotsopoulos J, Lubinski J, Neuhausen SL, *et al.* Hormone replacement therapy and the risk of ovarian cancer in *BRCA1* and *BRCA2* mutation carriers. *Gynecol Oncol* 2006;**100**:83–8.

Mascarenhas C, Lambe M, Bellocco R, *et al.* Use of hormone replacement therapy before and after ovarian cancer diagnosis and ovarian cancer survival. *Int J Cancer* 2006;**119**:2907–15.

McDonnell BA, Twiggs LB. Hormone replacement therapy in endometrial cancer survivors: new perspectives after the heart and estrogen progestin replacement study and the women's health initiative. *J Low Genit Tract Dis* 2006;**10**:92–101.

Pothuri B, Ramondetta L, Martino M, *et al.* Development of endometrial cancer after radiation treatment for cervical carcinoma. *Obstet Gynecol* 2003;**101**:941–5.

Ursic-Vrscaj M, Bebar S, Zakelj MP. Hormone replacement therapy after invasive ovarian serous cystadenocarcinoma treatment: the effect on survival. *Menopause* 2001;**8**:70–5.

Other cancers

Kennelly R, Kavanagh DO, Hogan AM, Winter DC. Oestrogen and the colon: potential mechanisms for cancer prevention. *Lancet Oncol* 2008;**9**:385–91.

La Vecchia C, Gallus S, Fernandez E. Hormone replacement therapy and colorectal cancer: an update. *J Br Menopause Soc* 2005;**11**:166–72.

Prihartono N, Palmer JR, Louik C, *et al.* A case-control study of use of postmenopausal female hormone supplements in relation to the risk of large bowel cancer. *Cancer Epidemiol Biomarkers Prev* 2000;**9**:443–7.

Naldi L, Altieri A, Imberti GL, *et al.* Cutaneous malignant melanoma in women. Phenotypic characteristics, sun exposure, and hormonal factors: a case-control study from Italy. *Ann Epidemiol* 2005;**15**:545–50.

Persson I, Yuen J, Bergkvist L, Schairer C. Cancer incidence and mortality in women receiving estrogen and estrogen-progestin replacement therapy – long-term follow-up of a Swedish cohort. *Int J Cancer* 1996;**67**:327–32.

Rossouw JE, Anderson GL, Prentice RL, *et al.*; Writing Group for the Women's Health Initiative Investigators. Risks and benefits of estrogen plus progestin in healthy postmenopausal women: principal results from the Women's Health Initiative randomized controlled trial. *JAMA* 2002;**288**:321–33.

Smith MA, Fine JA, Barnhill RL, Berwick M. Hormonal and reproductive influences and risk of melanoma in women. *Int J Epidemiol* 1998;**27**:751–7.

Index

Page references to *figures, tables and text boxes* are shown in *italics*.
Reports, studies and trials have been grouped together under studies.